T0354744

GO!GO!GO!

RISE, FALL, AND RISE AGAIN: THE STORY OF CANCER

Rob Atteberry

 iUniverse®

GO! GO! GO!
RISE, FALL, AND RISE AGAIN: THE STORY OF CANCER

iUniverse books may be ordered through booksellers or by contacting:

iUniverse
1663 Liberty Drive
Bloomington, IN 47403
www.iuniverse.com
1-800-Authors (1-800-288-4677)

ISBN: 978-1-5320-2314-9 (sc)
ISBN: 978-1-5320-2315-6 (e)

Library of Congress Control Number: 2017909053

Print information available on the last page.

iUniverse rev. date: 06/15/2017

To my sons,
Max, Wes, Ben, and Zac,
I hope this book leads you each to live your best life.

My wife,
Keri,
I love you. You are the world to me.

My dad and mom,
Max and Diane,
I love you.

My family and friends,
your constant love and support mean everything to me.

My doctors,
thank you for your meticulous care.

Cancer fighters and survivors everywhere,
never give up!

God,
thank you for each and every precious day.

Steve Ryman,
thank you for being a friend and for
inspiring me to write this book.

CONTENTS

AUTHOR'S NOTE

Our sense of hearing can transport us back to a different time, place, or experience. For this reason, music is often linked to our memories. How often have you found yourself driving down the highway when an old tune comes on the radio and you instinctively raise the volume? Do you have a specific playlist that you listen to while working out because it invigorates and motivates you? If that one special song is played at a friend's wedding, do you and your spouse exchange a knowing glance before taking the dance floor? Hearing certain songs can excite us, make us melancholy, and remind us of specific times in our lives.

Since music has always been an important part of my life and an integral part of my relationship with my wife, Keri, it seemed appropriate that I use meaningful song titles to name chapters of my story.

In this book, you'll come to know both halves of my duet and our own little quartet. You'll witness firsthand my song with all its scores, adagio moments, ever-changing tempo, staccato sidebars, and refrains that have led me to know the greatest Maestro of this thing called life as I gratefully play my encore.

PROLOGUE

The exhaustion hung on me like a heavy, wet blanket I couldn't lift. Although I slept much, I never felt rested; I wondered whether I would ever feel rested again. The new me was nothing like the person I'd been only a few months before, when my focus had been meeting deadlines and surpassing goals to hit weekly, monthly, and quarterly numbers.

My reflection in the mirror bore little resemblance to the fit guy who'd once been an overachiever, competed in triathlons, and chased after personal bests both at work and at home. Gone were the toned biceps and defined shoulders I'd honed over years of swimming; the eager eyes that took on any project—big or small; and the ready grin that made strangers into friends. Gone, too, were the strong arms that had protected my wife and rocked my sons; gone were the solid thighs that had characterized me as a cyclist and runner.

Who are you? I thought.

As I looked at the man in the mirror, I wondered whether I'd ever again see the hardworking guy who could always deliver and get the job done, no questions asked and no matter the sacrifice. Higher sales, lower expenses, less shrink, more profits—whatever the target, I'd deliver. It was just who I was; I'd built a great career by working harder and longer than the next guys, and I had no complaints.

Where is that *guy?* I wondered as I realized I missed him.

The guy in the mirror had eyes vaguely similar to mine, yet my mind didn't want to believe they were my own. They looked dull, tired, and void of their eager glimmer. It seemed so long ago that I'd dutifully left home each morning and returned late at night, often after the kids had eaten dinner and taken their baths. Back then I eagerly did it all over again the next morning, after just a few hours of sleep.

The pace had been nonstop, the goals never ending, and I liked it. I thought it was how things were supposed to be. I liked my busy, goal-driven life, and I liked building a comfortable lifestyle for our family. I liked that other guy who used to meet me at the mirror. I'd been proud of all he'd achieved. When I'd met him at the mirror in days gone by, in the early-morning hours long before the sun came up, he had a familiar, eager, can-do attitude. I liked that guy's style, character, and ethics.

But where did he go?

The stranger's tired eyes that stared back at me were framed by a patchy, distorted face with flakes of peeling skin in various stages of healing. I studied the haphazard palette of reds, pinks, oranges, and purples that marred his sallow complexion. His ravaged face looked pained. I studied how sickening colors framed a sunken, gray-blue pallor beneath listless, tired eyes.

The apathetic stranger looked like he'd survived a terrible and life-altering event. I studied the reflection a little longer, turning my head to examine a new patch of raw skin that had scabbed over since the day before.

At least it's healing, I reminded myself.

While most of my hair had been gone for some time, and I really didn't miss it, the burned, peeling, scabby skin was unattractive, to say the least. If my sense of smell hadn't been diminished, I'd have smelled the sickening, putrid odor of burned skin and hair that's so distinct and repugnant, usually an unwelcome reminder of a horrific accident.

But my condition hadn't resulted from an accident. The treatments had been ordered and efficiently scheduled. I'd gone willingly to have them administered one by one, and the poison had rhythmically dripped into my veins, one drop at a time.

The painful burning sensation, deadened taste buds, loss of sense of smell, and itchy, flaky patches of skin had all been expected—certainly not welcomed, but expected nonetheless. My rational side reminded me that the guy in the mirror was only a temporary visitor. The fatigue, pain, unsightliness, and discomfort were small prices to pay to still be here with Keri and the boys. I shook off the thought of the other possibility.

Reminded of our boys, I went to join them outside, and I heard their voices become louder as I stepped out the door. Smiling, I stood and watched our firstborn son while he played in the yard with his brothers. Instantly I was reminded that it had all been worth it and that I'd endure it all again in a heartbeat.

Being literally cooked from the inside out has certainly been worth it, I thought. *To be here with—with—*

The tallest boy I watched was most definitely my firstborn and one of my greatest sources of pride and joy on this earth. I could see his name in my mind's eye, but it wouldn't come to me. *Why can't I say his name? Why can't I remember how to say the name of my own son?*

My stomach felt queasy again, so I went back inside, through our home's side entrance, and into the mudroom. There was *his* jacket, and there were *his* shoes haphazardly tossed on the floor like always, waiting for *him*—waiting for—for—

I wracked my brain and willed myself to put together the letters to call up his name. My mind rapidly searched its memory banks again and again. I began to sweat. Anxiety welled within my chest, nausea washed over me, and my heart raced uncontrollably. I just couldn't make the connection, no matter how hard I tried. I knew my son's name, yet my brain wouldn't combine the letters or send the word to my mouth so I could *say* it. I slumped against the doorframe as Keri came near.

"What is it? Rob, what's wrong?" she asked.

With tears in my eyes and a sickening feeling in the pit of my stomach, I shook my head as if to rattle loose the simplest yet most important syllables that no father could possibly forget how to utter. His name," I said, with tears in my eyes. "It's like I know it, but I can't form it and say it! I can't remember how to *say* his *name*—my own son's name, Keri—the son we named after my dad."

Keri hugged me and held on to me as tears fell down my face and onto my shirt. "Max, honey. It's Max," she said as she rubbed my back and held me close.

1

To Be Young

By Ryan Adams

O urs had always been a fairly traditional marriage, and we had a household not unlike many others inside the comfortable family homes that lined our manicured street. I had married the love of my life, and I'd known Keri since she was eight and I was twelve. Although we'd known one another as kids, it wasn't until my first year out of college that we started to date.

Keri was sixteen and I was twenty when we both had summer jobs as lifeguards at the Great Oaks Country Club. My dad's job had brought our family back to Rochester, Michigan. I first met Keri when we were on the swim team as kids. Lifeguarding was a natural fit for me, as I'd been in the pool for years by then. Keri caught my eye when I saw her again at the country club pool where we both worked as lifeguards. But since she was still sixteen, I didn't think I should ask her out—yet. Working together during five-hour shifts at the pool gave us plenty of time to get to know one another. There was nothing we didn't talk about in those days.

After attending Miami University in Ohio, I moved back to

1

Rochester in my third year of college. Keri and I were dating other people at the time, and our friend groups sometimes did things together, which frequently put us in the same situations. I was still drawn to her infectious smile, and I quickly decided she was the nicest person I'd ever met. Before long, I couldn't stop thinking of "cute Keri."

Things eventually fell into place for us, and Keri and I began to see each other when she was eighteen. She was at Michigan State, and I was working in Muskegon, but we drove to visit each other all the time. After our first date, we were basically inseparable.

Keri and I dated for five years, and we became very close. One of the main things we had in common was our love of music. Even in our earlier days of lifeguarding, she and I talked about and bonded over music. We spent hours making mixtapes for each other and sharing songs.

When I asked Keri to marry me three years into our relationship, I gave her a mixtape I'd made of special songs. Music had always been an important part of our lives and our relationship, and it continued to be important over the years. When I gave her the mixtape, Keri knew I'd carefully selected each song especially for her.

After a two-year engagement, Keri and I married in 2000, with all our friends and family at our wedding celebration. I was thrilled to walk into our future together, side by side with the cutest, coolest, and nicest girl. Our future was bright, and we looked forward to our new life together.

Before we married, I was an area sales manager with Elder-Beerman Department Stores. In my first position with them, I oversaw three area managers and thirty to forty associates. While I was one of the youngest managers in the company, I was good at my job, and I excelled quickly—just like I thought I was supposed to and just like I'd always envisioned I would do in my career.

In 1996, I took a position with the Gechsmin Corporation as a logistics analyst, and I steadily moved up the ranks, a year at a time. By 1999, I began traveling overseas several times a year on business trips for a couple of weeks at a time. Sometimes I went to Germany or China; I also made monthly trips to Las Vegas, Chicago, New York, Los Angeles, or Florida to attend shows. It was the nature of my job, and I enjoyed the pace and the responsibility of being the face of the company. In no time, I was a Delta Platinum member, thanks to all the miles I flew.

With my career going well, I knew it was time to take another step forward in my life plan. When I married Keri in 2000, everything in my world seemed right. I diligently steered my career and met my personal and professional goals. I was on top of the world.

Marrying Keri was another step in having my life fall into place as I pursued our happily-ever-after. Things were working out in my career and my personal life just as I'd planned. Like many men, I had a vision of the American dream in my mind's eye, and I looked toward the nice suburban home and a houseful of children.

After our two-week Hawaiian honeymoon, I dutifully plunged into my job as a buyer for Gechsmin's Home Division, a position I'd held for about a year by this time. During our honeymoon, I kept in touch with the office and handled issues from my laptop.

I'm sure Keri wasn't thrilled about it, but she knew how tenacious I'd always been in my work.

As newlyweds, Keri and I lived in Rochester for three years. Our first son was born and spent the first eight months of his life there. I focused on my job, determined to climb the corporate ladder and to get ahead in life as fast as I could. The hours were many, but I had a great boss, Paula Paquette, and I was surrounded by awesome people. I thoroughly enjoyed my job, and for eight years I thrived on delivering results.

The long hours and personal sacrifices seemed normal to me as I rose within the company's ranks. By 2001, when I was just twenty-nine, I was named vice president of the Soft Home division. I loved what I did. I'd even go so far as to say it exhilarated and energized me to oversee a sales volume of more than $2 billion and a staff of twelve, which included six buyers. Responsible for the company's bedding, bath, window, kitchen textiles, and floor categories, I developed the Thalia brand in Soft Home that focused heavily on the Hispanic demographic. As a divisional vice president, I expanded our Martha Stewart brand and introduced new products. I also reintroduced the line's three-, four-, and five-star bed-and-bath products.

While I worked hard to get ahead for Keri and me, we were blessed with our first child, Max, who was born in 2002 and was instantly the light of our life. Our newly expanded young family lived in a nice condo in Rochester. With my dad's help, we worked hard together for many months to renovate the condo, and it was perfect for us at the time.

For the first three months after Max's birth, Keri continued her work as a first-grade teacher. We were fortunate to have our parents help us care for little Max, but Keri and I both eventually decided that she should stay home with our new son.

Life couldn't have been better, from where I stood. I had a beautiful wife, a precious new son. and a great career, There was a lot happening in our lives, and I enjoyed the pulse and pace of it. It felt like the puzzle pieces were falling into place and that Keri and I were on our way to creating the perfect American dream.

Before long, I was promoted to divisional vice president of Soft Home and Hard Home with Gechsmin. Max was walking, talking, and discovering his new world, and I was working hard to broaden my own horizons in order to give my family the life they deserved. It felt good to be our family's provider, and it was a role I relished.

By 2003, I was managing both the Soft and Hard Home teams, and was responsible for direct reports of buying and indirect reports of finance, advertising, and store operations. With ten buying teams—each comprising twenty or more team members, including two merchandising managers—I was responsible for a $3 billion segment of the company. Happily ensconced in my fast-paced corporate career, I also managed the $1.2 billion Martha Stewart Home brand for the company, with responsibilities that included brand development, marketing efforts, and in-store presentations, among countless other things.

When handled correctly, retail means revenues, and revenues mean dollars for everyone in the company. It was the perfect cause-and-effect example of how hard work and dedication pay off. It made sense, and it worked well with plans for my family's lifestyle and my own career path. I did my job, and I did it well.

I continued to rise within the corporate ranks at a young age. Everything was working out according to my plan, and I had the world by the tail, as far as I was concerned. My future looked bright and hopeful from where I stood in those early days. Only the sky seemed to be the limit, and I was determined to keep growing and improving as I built my career.

In less than a year as a divisional vice president, Gechsmin promoted me again, this time to vice president/GMM of Home and Home Electronics. As the title and the salary grew, so did the responsibilities and the workload. I was managing a $5 billion sales volume and overseeing eighteen buying teams with over forty team members and three divisional merchandise managers. I thrived in that high-pressure atmosphere, and I enjoyed that my progress was measurable and marked; in just one year, I had increased our gross margin and reduced inventory costs by 20 percent. My efforts were clearly reflected in their effects, and I liked being in control of the company's progress and contributing to its growth.

I was prepared to put in the work and the time to keep moving ahead. The corporate ladder held such promise, and I liked the idea that I was in control of my destiny and that life was working out just as it should.

2
Begin the Begin

By REM

While my corporate responsibilities increased, so did my results, and Gechsmin wasn't the only corporation to notice. After just a year in my vice-president role with Gechsmin, another hypermarket giant recruited me. Founded in 1934 as a supermarket, but later credited with pioneering the supercenter concept in 1962, Tendlart was a major player in the retail world. When they recruited me, Tendlart was on its way to becoming one of America's largest private companies and one of North America's top food retailers. The work ethic of Tendlart's founder, Hendrik Tendlart, a Dutch immigrant, mirrored my own.

I eagerly accepted Tendlart's offer to be a vice president and resigned from Gechsmin on good terms and with notice. The only negative thing about the job was that I had to move to Grand Rapids and into an apartment, while Keri and Max stayed behind for eight months. But Keri and I were a team, and we each did what we had to do to make things work.

In my position with Tendlart, I was responsible for

merchandising strategy and personnel development for the do-it-yourself, automotive, garden, pets and electronics/media teams. I jumped into my role with enthusiasm and worked harder than ever with my eye on the prize: to make a great life for our family.

Since I'd known at the time that Gechsmin would be moving its headquarters, and we didn't want to leave our Michigan family, Keri and I felt the Tendlart offer had come at a good time. She did her part and took care of Max and our home while I concentrated on my new role with Tendlart.

We moved to Ada, a suburb outside of Grand Rapids, when Max was two and a half. Things seemed nearly perfect. We were still close enough that Keri and I could see our families and friends on the weekends, and Keri stayed home and took care of Max. It felt like we were building our American dream, and I liked the idea that I was providing an ideal life for my family, as I'd always wanted to do.

My twelve-hour workdays became the norm. Keri never complained about having to shoulder the bulk of the parenting responsibilities, and we fell into the traditional roles of provider and caretaker. I took care of our finances and stability and handled the big picture, while Keri managed "home and hearth," taking care of the day-to-day details for our family. It was an exhilarating time, and I basked in my responsibilities.

Our families and friends have always been important to Keri and me, so we saw them every week, even after we'd moved to Grand Rapids. We wanted Max to grow up surrounded by family and good influences. It was all part of our traditional expectations and our own upbringings.

Many days—and nights—I focused on my job with Tendlart. I was responsible for fourteen buying teams of over sixty team members, which included three merchandise managers. It exhilarated me to manage over $1.1 billion in sales and to work with others to better their own careers as I furthered mine. My employees, my boss, my company, and my family all relied on me for results, and that was perfectly fine with me.

In my mind, I was doing what was expected of me and what was required to secure a good life. I'd never shied away from hard work, and I continued to push and push toward bigger, higher goals. I wasn't certain where my efforts would lead, but I was prepared to go the distance, no matter what.

Keri and I were thrilled when we learned she was pregnant with our second child. We were at a good place in our lives, and it was a good time to add to our family. In 2006, Wes joined our family, and Keri and I were thrilled that Max, three and a half by that time, had a little brother.

With a newborn and an active toddler, Keri had her hands full at home. We made a great team, though both of us were tired each night by the time we dropped into bed. Since she knew I had to be at work early in the morning, Keri always got up with Wes for his nighttime feedings and diaper changes. She was a natural mother, and she made it look easy. Having her at home with our boys made it easy for me to go to work and focus on my corporate responsibilities. I knew I was a lucky man—and for so many reasons.

About a year after Wes was born, Tendlart asked me to take over in 2007 as vice president of home and electronics and media. I was up for the challenge, and I plunged headfirst into my new position: merchandising strategies and personnel development of the Home areas.

With sixteen teams of seventy people and three merchandise managers, I was responsible for $1 billion in volume. While some people consider that too much pressure, I loved it. Within three years, I'd established strategic principles for pricing, marketing, store presentation, brands, and merchandise assortment across all business groups in my division. By 2010, the results of my efforts were once again measurable in increased year-over-year sales figures and a gain in market share that showed Tendlart had outpaced other retailers in the electronics industry for three years in a row.

While Keri managed our family and our home life, I managed the development and negotiation of multiple private-label programs. As Keri handled the needs of our boys, I handled my employees and my corporate responsibilities. She and I were a team, each managing our own parts of the equation.

With Max was in kindergarten and Wes as only a year old, we learned our family would be expanding again. Keri had her first ultrasound halfway through her pregnancy, at twenty weeks, and I was with her.

The ultrasound technician applied the sticky gel to Keri's abdomen and then moved the probe across her skin as she looked at the screen. Her eyes got bigger, and Keri and I looked at each other.

"What is it?" I asked. "Everything okay with the baby?"

"Have you had a previous ultrasound?" asked the technician.

Since we hadn't, Keri and I looked at each other with worried expressions, afraid something might be wrong with the baby.

"Well, you're having *twins!*"

"Ummm—what?" Keri asked.

She and I took deep breaths and tried to absorb what we'd heard. We were overwhelmed and extremely surprised. Of course, they were both boys.

I think Keri was numb with shock as the technician wiped off the sticky gel and helped her to sit up again. She and I didn't say much as we walked out of the obstetrician's office.

"Hungry?" I asked as we walked to our car.

"Of course. Let's get some pizza. Apparently, I'm eating for three!"

A few minutes later, Keri and I sat across from each other at a pizzeria. We just stared at each other as our new reality sunk in. It was a lot to absorb.

"Twins," she said.

"Yeah. Wow. At least we know how to raise boys already."

"What—are—we—gonna—do?" Keri said.

Then we both burst out laughing. We knew we'd be just fine.

Everyone's eyes got big when we told them we had not one but *two* more boys on the way. "Are you guys trying to start your own basketball team?" friends joked.

Throughout her pregnancy with the twins, Keri still managed our household and our two small boys. She was awesome, and I appreciated how she kept everything together so I could focus on my work.

By the time Ben and Zac came along in 2008, Keri had really learned to multitask. While she made it all seem easy, it would be some time before I realized the impact it was having on her.

3
I'm Ready

By Twin Shadow

W hile I put in eighty to one hundred hours a week at work, Keri held down the fort. We had a wonderful sitter, Abby, to help Keri with the boys' evening routines and give her a slight break, though taking care of four boys under the age of five was still a lot. Abby was the cousin of a neighbor and a college student when she began to help with the boys. She was an amazing help and quickly became part of our family.

As I'd leave for work in the mornings, Keri would ask, "So, do you think we'll see you before eight tonight? Maybe we can all eat dinner together."

"I'll try, but I never know how the day will play out," I'd answer as I kissed her goodbye.

My workdays didn't end when I left the office. Deadlines, figures, and issues still swirled around my head as if part of my makeup. When we had all the kids in the car, such as on the way to dinner or to visit family, the boys knew they were to keep quiet while I was on a business call.

It was Abby who helped Keri with dinner and bath time for the boys. I missed out on those as well as story time and rocking the boys to sleep, as I dutifully did what I thought I was supposed to do as a dad and a husband. Years later I learned that Keri had dressed newborn Max in cute little outfits every day at five in hopes that Daddy would be home to see him.

But Keri never complained. She was my support system and the reason I was able to rise in the ranks. Looking back, I think we each expected things to slow down and normalize in time. But the clock was ticking, and the calendar pages kept flipping as my boys grew up. I controlled aspects of my professional world, but I had no control over how quickly time passed.

When the boys started playing soccer and swimming, Keri drove them to practices. I made it to their games and meets, but I was *that dad* who was always dressed in business clothes, had a cell phone to his ear, and paced on the sidelines.

"Dad! Dad! Did you see it, Dad?" one of them would ask excitedly after a game. "Did you see me score?"

"Yeah, buddy! That was awesome!" I'd say, as I covered the mouthpiece of the phone that was still glued to my ear.

Even if I had to travel in late December, I always made it home for Christmas. But as Keri busily cooked dinner in the kitchen, I was often on my cell phone, cloistered away in my home office, dealing with work-related issues. Again, I felt I was doing what I had to do and what was expected of me.

I loved my boys more than anything and would do anything in the world for them, but Keri at times insisted I give the boys their baths or help them with their reading. It wasn't that she wanted me to do it; rather, she wanted to give me the experience of doing it before the opportunity was lost.

My dad had been the same. He'd always been the main breadwinner and the parent who went out and worked while Mom raised the kids. It seemed to me that if I worked and brought in a huge salary for my family, I was meeting expectations and fulfilling my role. But Keri was sort of a single parent at times. As much as I wanted the boys to call for me, it was *Mommy* who they called out for if they had a nightmare or a scraped knee and who they wanted to put Band-Aids on their injuries. It's all they'd known.

I later learned that Keri wasn't thrilled. She'd grown envious of some of the other women in our neighborhood whose husbands arrived home by five thirty like clockwork every evening.

My boys were growing up and becoming mannerly, articulate, and smart. Yet it was Mom who had swaddled them, taught them, soothed them, and guided them in their early years. It was Mom who had helped with homework, celebrated lost teeth, refereed squabbles, soothed hurt feelings, and dealt with the allergies that afflicted all of our boys.

While Keri handled the parenting at home, I was ensconced in my corporate world at Tendlart, and many changes were going on within the eighty-year-old company. Unlike Gechsmin, with its more than three thousand stores and corporate atmosphere, Tendlart had grown to 160 stores, one at a time, by the time I came onboard. Tendlart didn't have the infrastructure I'd grown accustomed to at Gechsmin. That was what I brought to Tendlart in the Home and Hard Lines areas. My mission was to make Electronics the best in the area and to anchor it with a solid Photo Processing section. I understood the company's strengths and weaknesses, and I knew what it needed from me and what I could contribute.

I had a great counterpart in Ruth, and although my boss was nice enough to me, he had a reputation for not being nice to all the other employees. He was an intense guy with a passion for Excel spreadsheets, and he loved his PowerPoint presentations. He expected all his people to be prepared for the company's Monday-morning meetings and to show up armed with their individual twenty-page reports, even if the reports had consumed their entire weekend.

Everyone in the company knew that he expected everyone to fall into step with him, no questions asked, no excuses accepted. That's just how he was. Even if I didn't agree with his management strategy or his tactics, I was a company guy, so I delivered at all costs, despite the constant stress.

My boss also had a reputation for being a talker and for never letting others get a word in edgewise. He loved his graphs, charts, and reports, and he was a paperwork guy who insisted on having things done his way. I imagined his entire life was charted on the spreadsheets he loved so much. He was three years older than I, and I sometimes saw him at the gym. He and I even worked out together a few times.

Our company president called me one day and said, "Look,

Rob, I know the guy is tough." He was one of those managers who presumed his job was to identify all the negatives, find fault, and call attention to problems. If there weren't any, he'd create some. So I spent a lot of time dealing with my boss's idiosyncrasies and time-wasting requirements.

Things had become very tenuous at work when my boss came onboard, and they only became worse. I knew he didn't particularly like me, but his boss, the company president, liked me—and we were friends.

By this time, I'd begun to feel the stress, and it had begun to affect my sleep. Coupled that with a sinus irritation, and I spent most nights tossing and turning and trying to get comfortable in a position that allowed me to breathe. Each night, as soon as I lay down, I noticed my sinuses felt congested, and the battle for sleep began. When the alarm went off each morning, I dragged myself from our bed and into the shower so I could wake up and start the cycle all over again.

I felt tired most of the time, but since I hadn't been sleeping well, I attributed it to the lack of sleep. I'd also begun to get frequent nosebleeds that came on quickly, with no warning, and lasted quite a while.

One night, while at the movies with Keri, I suddenly got a nosebleed. While she ran to get some napkins for me, I wondered why the nosebleeds seemed to be happening more and more often. She and I had presumed it must be the result of whatever sinus condition afflicted me. I stopped the bleeding and went on with life as usual.

After eight years with Tendlart—and no telling how much precious family time and the boys' "firsts" forever lost—our company president called me into his office one day. What happened next came was a shock. For the first time in my life, I was unceremoniously let go from my job.

That afternoon, I told Bruce, the president of Hydeswort Companies, whom I'd known from Gechsmin. "Sure!" he said. "Come on over, and we can walk the place and talk about a possible VP position for you."

A week later, I met with him in Detroit and was hired. Relationships, networking, and my reputation had paid off for me.

4
Something's Wrong

By Sloan

I was eager to jump into my new job with Hydeswort Companies, America's leading manufacturer and marketer of outdoor cushions, furniture, and décor. I was based out of its corporate office in Detroit in my new position as vice president of new business development. The logistics meant Keri and the boys lived in Grand Rapids while I lived with my parents in Detroit. It wasn't an ideal situation, but once again, Keri and I worked as a team, each of us handling our specific responsibilities to make things work.

As always, I plunged headfirst into my new role, intently focused on getting results and making a name for myself with Hydeswort. I immediately established a new business team, implemented a new product process to be used across the company for future business ideas, and developed and implemented new market strategies for the company. With nearly two decades of experience in retail management and executive administration, I was in my element and energized by the prospects of my future with the company.

While I was busy with my corporate life, working twelve hours a day and making buying trips to China, Keri continued to take care of our four boys at home. I was approaching my fortieth birthday, and it felt like I had the perfect life on all fronts.

The only thing that hindered me in the slightest was the nagging sinus infection that had started well over a year earlier and had followed me from Tendlart to Hydeswort. I'd taken all the usual over-the-counter sinus medications, and I saw a doctor who prescribed some antibiotics, but nothing seemed to lessen the symptoms.

I felt worse at nighttime, when I had trouble breathing and couldn't sleep well. When I competed in a triathlon, along with a friend, my sinus infection made it hard to breathe. I'd completed many triathlons, so I knew it was unusual for me to feel that way.

"I wonder when this infection will clear up," I said to Keri one night after I'd come home late from work. "I've never had a cold or sinus problem that hung on for so long."

"Well, I bought you a new hypoallergenic allergy pillow today," she said. "I think maybe you've got allergies instead of a sinus infection. It's worth a try."

But the new allergy pillow made no difference. I still couldn't sleep, and as a result, I didn't feel rested during the workday. The longer this went on, the worse I felt. I was approaching forty, so I assumed I was just getting a little older and perhaps I needed to get more exercise to improve my sleep quality. I was certain that whatever afflicted me had a simple explanation. I just hoped I'd feel better for my birthday celebration, which was coming up in a few months.

We enjoyed a great Christmas 2011 with our boys and our families, and we looked toward to the promise of the new year. I felt tired, but I figured my nonstop work life was just catching up with me and I simply needed some rest. That nagging sinus infection had never gone away, so I still wasn't sleeping well at night.

Just six days into 2012, I'd had enough of feeling lousy, and Keri took me to the emergency room. The doctor examined me, told me that something had been going around, and prescribed more antibiotics with instructions to take all the medication, drink plenty of fluids, and use a humidifier at night when I slept.

As the seasons changed, and we went into springtime, I still had gotten no relief, and the doctors continued to diagnose acute rhinitis and acute maxillary sinusitis. They prescribed still more antibiotics, steroids for the inflammation, and nasal inhalers.

"Drink plenty of water," the doctors reminded me. "And get lots of rest."

Keri made all the arrangements for my fortieth birthday. Somehow, between juggling all her responsibilities of mothering four boys, including a set of twins, she put together an incredible celebration.

Family and friends have always been very important to me, with my love for music following close behind. Even though I didn't feel well, I was determined to enjoy my birthday surrounded by the people who meant the most to me.

When Saturday night came, a dozen couples, including our closest friends and family, joined us in downtown Detroit. Keri had set up everything in advance, including reserving hotel rooms at a casino. With friends, family, and music, it was sure to be the perfect birthday. Keri reserved a VIP area at a nightclub, but she'd expected we'd all gamble first at the casino and then go to the nightclub as a secondary option. As it turned out, our fun, eclectic group danced in the nightclub till three in the morning.

My sister, Cindy, made my birthday cake shaped like an old-style Atari console—something that only people of my generation would recognize. It felt very good to turn forty surrounded by the people I loved. Life was good, and the future seemed even brighter when I shut my eyes and held my wife after we'd partied the night away. It felt like I had it all. Life was coming together just as I wanted.

So life was terrific from where I stood—except for that nagging sinus condition I just couldn't shake. I'd had a CT scan done a week before my party, so Keri and I assumed we'd soon have some answers. I figured my doctor would simply change my medication, and I'd soon be well.

Living in two different households was far from ideal—for any of us. But we knew it was just a temporary arrangement since the boys needed to complete the school year in Grand Rapids. Keri and I didn't like it, but we made it work from different sides of the state.

Just days before I'd turned forty, I went on a buying trip to China. Already worn down from the longtime lack of sleep, my nagging sinus condition made the trip miserable. I'd been on various medications by this time and had recently been treated for bronchitis.

I knew I'd receive the results from the CT scan that had been done before my birthday party, and I hoped they'd provide some answers. I had previously sought the opinion of another doctor, Dr. Bowman, and he had ordered the CT scan of my sinuses to better identify the problem. Keri and I felt hopeful that we'd finally get some answers so I could get better and get on with my life. More than anything, I wanted to feel better and more rested.

On the day of the scan, as I waited for the technician to complete the images, my mind had been on some issues at work, and I was eager to get back there. Just taking time from work for the CT scan had aggravated me. But I knew the scan would pinpoint the stubborn infection that had plagued me for months.

Back from my China trip, I was driving and preoccupied with thoughts of an upcoming meeting when my cell phone rang. It was the doctor, and he told me the CT scan results. I tried to steady myself, but it was like I'd been kicked in the stomach. I tried to catch my breath. "Yes, okay. Thank you, Doctor," I numbly replied as I hung up.

It suddenly seemed so cruel—to both of us—that Keri was

hundreds of miles away when I got the news. I just had to talk to her as I tried to digest what I'd just heard.

As I shakily dialed my cell phone, it all seemed surreal, as if I were an observer looking at the life of someone else who had just been dealt the blow of a lifetime. It couldn't possibly be *my* life or *my family's* life that would be affected by what I'd just heard. I was a husband, a father, and a busy executive with responsibilities, deadlines, and projects to complete. My life was going great, and I was building a life for my family. I simply had no time for such things as what the doctor had described.

I thought, *We were all just happily celebrating my birthday and without a care in the world. Life looked so perfect and promising that night! How can all of it change in the blink of eye?*

"Hey!" Keri cheerfully answered when I called, and I heard splashing and children's voices in the background that told me she was at swim practice with Max.

"It's a tumor! It's a tumor!" I screamed as the reality began to sink in for me.

I'm usually excitable, so this reaction seemed normal to Keri. She'd been expecting my call. She was silent, but I could feel her shock on the other end, as if she were right next to me in the room.

I learned later that as she sat poolside next to a girlfriend at Max's swim practice, she'd tried to absorb the news calmly and keep it together as I screamed the word *tumor* over and over. She told me later that it broke her heart that she couldn't hold me and hug me in that moment as she wrestled to find something reassuring to say while her own heart was breaking.

"But it's probably benign, right?" Keri eagerly asked as she tried to stay positive. "I'm sure it'll be benign, Rob."

"They'll know when they get in there and have a better look. They're scheduling me for a biopsy."

I focused on my work as I waited for the biopsy date to come. I wanted nothing more than to have the tumor removed and to hear that it was nothing to worry about. The doctor, however, explained that he'd intended to biopsy only a part of the tumor as the first step.

Two weeks later, my mother-in-law went to stay with the boys so Keri could be with me in Rochester for the surgery.

Keri kissed me one last time before the gowned nurses rolled me into the surgery unit where the biopsy would be performed.

"It'll be fine," she said with a smile. "I love you."

"Love you too! See you soon."

The doctor went out to speak to Keri a little while later. She eagerly got up and walked to meet him, and my parents and my sister followed her too. As he removed his scrubs cap from his head, he said, "Well, I went ahead and removed it while I was in there. The tissue appears bloody and soft. Just looking at it, I don't think it'll be cancer, but we'll send it off just to be sure."

Keri drove me back to my parents' condo the day before Mother's Day and stayed by my side while I was on my back for the next twenty-four hours, per my doctor's orders. It felt odd to be together in the master bedroom of that condo because it had been ours before we sold it to my parents. The surroundings were oddly familiar, yet Keri and I had grown so much and gone through so many changes since we'd lived there.

Two weeks later, Keri and I were laughing and joking when we walked into my doctor's office to get the results. The nurse showed us to an exam room, where I sat on the exam table and Keri took a seat in a chair across from me and against a wall.

The doctor walked in as we were laughing about something one of the boys had done. His face looked somber, and he held a clipboard in front of him. I studied his face yet had no clue what he'd say to us.

He took a deep breath. "The results are in," he said. "And it's not the diagnosis I expected—not at all. It's lymphoma."

It felt like I'd been kicked in the stomach as the doctor's words plunged into me. Keri covered her mouth. Just the suffix *oma* meant *cancer,* and it was the one thing we hadn't expected to hear—not in a million years.

I took a deep breath and was ready to hear what we'd do about this obstacle that had been put in my path. As far as I was concerned, it was a hurdle I'd go over or even go through, but it wasn't going to block me forever.

"It'll be okay," the doctor told us as he turned to Keri and outlined what would happen next.

We walked out of the doctor's office and got in our car completely changed from the happy, carefree couple we'd been just an hour earlier when we'd walked in. Keri drove us home while I called my parents. After I dialed the phone, she reached over and held my hand as we drove through traffic.

How can I tell them this? I thought while I waited for them to pick up. I was a parent with sons of my own, and I could think of nothing worse to hear from one of them—no matter their age.

Dad didn't hear well over the phone, so I knew I'd have to speak loudly, which only made delivering the news more offensive and brutal. My heart raced, and I took a deep breath as I waited.

"Dad?" I said loudly.

"Rob! Hi!"

"Dad, I have cancer."

"What?" Dad asked.

"Dad, I have *cancer*!" I said louder.

I felt the words hit him through the phone. It seemed cruel to tell him my news. He'd always been the strong patriarch of our family, and he and Mom had always had positive attitudes, no matter what. I knew he'd paused to digest what he'd just heard.

"It'll be fine, Rob," he said after a short silence. "Everything's going to be fine."

I needed that. I needed Dad's strength and his positivity in that moment, just as I'd needed my dad for less significant problems over the years. He'd taken a little bit of the burden and put it on his own shoulders, just as he'd always done and just as we'd counted on him to do. Dad's shoulders were even bigger than I'd known.

Keri still held my hand, and she squeezed it as she drove us home. Sometimes words simply weren't needed, and this was one of those times. Our intertwined fingers said it all. I knew she would be with me for whatever lay ahead. For better or for worse, in sickness and in health, she'd be there.

5
Seasons

By Future Islands

The days continued to go by though, as did the seasons, while the world kept spinning. But with my cancer diagnosis came the reality that my fortieth birthday had been the last fun, carefree time I'd know for a long time—or maybe forever. There was "the time before," when everything seemed light, airy, and positive, and "the time after," when things were tenuous, scary, and dark.

My new world seemed uncertain and tentative as I realized how life could change drastically and in less than a week. I wished we could go back to my happy, carefree birthday celebration, surrounded by those who meant so much to me. I'd have given anything to go back to that innocent time before I knew about the nasty disease that could steal my life away and take me from Keri and the boys. How I wished we'd all been right when we thought I simply had allergies or a persistent sinus infection. We'd never imagined the worst—never in a million years.

The *C* word seemed so daunting and uncertain. But, as with

most things in life, I decided to create an orderly plan, work that plan, and get results. I drew strength from our family and friends, who all came through for us as I tackled cancer head-on.

When I began chemotherapy, Keri and the boys were still living in Grand Rapids, since the boys were still finishing school. The house we were having built in Clarkston was almost complete; we were set to move in one month. I was with my parents at their condo, and Keri's parents were keeping the boys for us so she could accompany me to the chemo treatments.

"You know you'd easily qualify to take leave your job under the FMLA laws," a friend told me.

"I can work through the chemo," I said with optimism. "I'll make it work. I can do it!"

Keri was at my side as the chemo drugs dripped through an IV into my body. Dr. Howard had explained how chemo works, and Keri and I had read online about it too. Knowledge is power, and I wanted to know how this part of my plan would work. We knew chemo worked to stop or slow the growth of cancer cells, which grow and divide quickly. However, while attacking the cancerous cells, they also harm healthy cells that divide quickly, especially those that line the mouth and intestines and cause hair to grow. Damage to the healthy cells can cause multiple side effects, some of which are very uncomfortable. I wasn't sure exactly what to expect, but I'd heard and read stories.

Thankfully, today's technology makes it easier and more

convenient to keep our family and friends updated on all that's going on in our world. People constantly called, sent e-mails, and texted to find out how I was doing. And Keri did her best to reply to them as we moved through our new journey. She checked in with everyone via a text message in the earliest days of our unwanted adventure:

> Hello everyone! Just had a chance to get back to all of you and let you know what's happening. Rob had a port put in, and he received a dose of chemo. He took it like a champ, though he felt a little nauseated. Rob's spirits are good, and his attitude is great, as usual. Thank you all for your thoughts and prayers!

Keri and I tried to stay positive, talking and joking with the nurses and each other as the invasive medicine dripped into my veins. While I waited for the session to end, my mind wandered to all the projects I'd been working on at the office. As vice president, I'd worked to establish the new business team, which included people in marketing, product management, social media, industrial design, and product design. I'd implemented a new product process to be used companywide for future business ideas. I'd also developed and implemented a new strategy for a first-to-market product in the outdoor products division that included legal, testing, sourcing, marketing, product development, and branding.

So my work life was busy, and there was so much going on I

hated to take time out for chemo treatments. One day, when Keri couldn't stay for the entire three-hour session, my sister, Cindy, came and sat with me. If indeed there's strength in numbers, the family did their best to lend me theirs as my own was challenged.

I quickly learned what to expect with the whole chemo process. We packed a cooler with Popsicles, cold drinks, and fruit. And as the chemo dripped into me, we passed the time by watching movies on my iPad. I knew that on day two following chemo I'd feel feverish and nauseated, so when the chemo sessions finished, I tried to get as much done at work as possible before the debilitating side effects struck.

One day, while at chemo, I looked around at the other people in the room with me. Seeing all the other cancer patients lined up in their chairs, with IVs dripping into their arms, I realized how prevalent cancer is and how it inflicts itself on unsuspecting people, interrupting lives, plans, and families. We all had our own agendas, families, hopes, and dreams, but we all shared one thing that united us. We'd placed our faith in our doctors, said our respective prayers, and desperately wanted to live for ourselves and for our families that needed us.

Cancer doesn't discriminate, as evidenced by people of all ages, from teenagers to the elderly, lined up around the chemo room that day. I wondered about all of them, their lives, their families, and their individual worlds. There was a pretty teenage girl who might have had cheerleading practice on any other day; an elderly gentleman whose white-haired wife sat beside him, holding his hand as she had probably done for half a century; a middle-aged Latina woman who talked on the phone about arrangements to pick up her kids from school; and all sorts of people of various ages and ethnicities. Each of them had lives, plans, dreams, and responsibilities, just like I did. I only hoped each of them also had a strong, loving family and devoted friends to support them and help them through the uncertain months that lay ahead.

The whole cancer thing had thrown a wrench in my orderly, responsible, and predictable world. But I knew it was something I had to deal with so I could again focus on my work. It would be an inconvenience, but I knew I'd get through it. I had to get through it. Keri and the boys were counting on me.

The first few chemo treatments went as well as could be expected. Our friends and family were our rocks during this time, pitching in and helping with the kids, accompanying me to chemo, coming to see me, and constantly keeping in touch.

I felt tired, of course—as if I had hardly any energy. My world didn't stop though, and work called to me. In the mornings, I had my coffee, tried to muster the energy needed just to get in my car, and dragged myself into my office. What I'd once done without thinking was now an exhausting chore. Even the simplest of tasks zapped my energy and left me feeling withered and wasted. I hardly knew the guy whose tired eyes looked at me from my car's rearview mirror.

My boss, Walter, was unlike any I'd had before. He'd been employed in eight jobs—versus the three I'd had—and I wonder why. When he moved me to another area of the office building, I thought he felt I threatened his position with the company. While I'd once worked on important projects with heavy responsibilities, my new role left me feeling unchallenged and as if I'd been given busy work that would be best suited to new hires. Walter reported to Bruce, and I got along well with him, but there was a chain of command to be respected, so I decided to bide my time and go along with Walter's whims.

Since I'd always been very detail oriented, I documented all my appointments and logged my meetings. In an effort to dutifully keep my employer updated, I sent an e-mail to Walter on July 11:

Quick reminder ... Next Monday, July 16th, I will be out of the office all day for Day One of the 2nd treatment of Chemo. On Day Two, Tuesday, July 17th, I'll need to leave by 2:30 for the second portion of the chemo. This treatment will be my 2nd out of 6 treatments, which will occur every three weeks. Approximately two weeks after the chemo is completed I will then begin 30 days of radiation. The plan is that cancer will be beaten, and all treatments will be complete by Halloween.

Thanks.

Rob Atteberry

6
Running up That Hill

By Kate Bush

With all that had been going on lately, Keri and I were crazy busy. We had moved into our new home on July 2, less than a month after I'd started chemo. Instead of being an exciting time, that summer seemed overwhelmingly busy as our family tried to settle into our new home while I battled cancer.

After a few weeks in our new home, we were still settling in. As if things couldn't get any more hectic and just when I was sure there was no chance of any worse news than I'd already gotten, we received a phone call on July 30. My dad's brother and my only blood-related uncle, Dale, had died of lung cancer.

"I've got to be in Missouri," I told Keri. "I've got to get to the funeral."

Keri had been getting the house organized while tending to my needs and caring for the boys, since I wasn't much help at that point. I don't know what I'd have done without her. "I'll drive you," she said. "We'll go to Missouri, and the boys can stay here with my parents."

"I'll let them know at work," I said as Keri went to get our suitcases.

My stomach felt queasy, and I was exhausted as I dialed my boss to tell him I'd need to be gone for a couple of days for the funeral.

"Rob, do you really need to go?" my boss asked.

I hesitated as the crassness of his question sank in, then replied, "Ah, yeah. Yes, I really do. Our family is very close; he's my only blood uncle, and I need to be there."

As Keri drove us to Missouri, I fielded phone calls from my office and my employees. She spent most of the time on her phone with my doctor as she tried to get a prescription sent to a Saint Louis pharmacy near where we'd be staying.

I was exhausted, but even worse were the painful sores all over the inside of my mouth. I'd dealt with mouth sores throughout my treatment, but this time it was much worse than ever before. It was incredibly painful to speak with thrush, or *candidiasis*, the fungal infection that had spread throughout my mouth, another side effect of the chemo. I was miserable as I took phone calls. While Keri drove, she handed me biotin gum to soothe and moisten my mouth, which was full of canker sores.

"Rob, you can't keep this up," Keri urged. "Just let the calls go to voice mail." But it would have bothered me not to respond and help people, since it was important for me to pull my weight, even with all I had going on.

As soon as we got to Saint Louis, Keri drove us straight to the pharmacy to pick up my prescription of liquid nystatin, the generic for Bio-Statin, which is an oral antifungal medication. We next went to the funeral home and then went to dinner with my family, although I could barely keep my eyes open by that time. My mom hadn't seen me in six weeks, because she and Dad had been at the lake, so she was utterly shocked by how much weight I'd lost and how sickly I looked. I was too weak and tired to talk about much of anything, and the mouth sores prevented me from even trying. I wanted nothing more than to get to the hotel and lie down.

When we got to the hotel later that night, I began to shake, possibly out of sheer exhaustion. The shaking had been happening frequently in the last few weeks, so Keri and I had developed a routine to help me get through it. She'd climb into bed with me, spoon my body with hers, and hold me tight until her body heat stopped the uncontrolled shivering. On that night, I fell asleep as Keri held me and kept me warm. This scene had become a routine with us because I couldn't control my own body temperature anymore.

Before dawn, I woke up and carefully got out of bed so as not to wake Keri. I grabbed my laptop and went to the desk in our hotel room.

Hours later, when the alarm went off, Keri woke up and asked, "Rob, what are you doing?"

"I've got to get this stuff done before we leave for the funeral this morning," I said.

"What? How long have you been up?"

"I don't know—maybe three hours. I just want to get this work done before we leave for the funeral."

"Here you go," Keri said as she wrapped a blanket around my shoulders.

"I just need another hour or so, and then I'll be done here," I said.

We attended my uncle's funeral, and as I looked around at all the mourners, I was even more convinced I'd dig in and fight my own cancer. It was too painful to think of Keri and our boys without me. I was even more determined to fight the beast that threatened not only me, but also our whole family. The chemo was miserable and the side effects daunting. But just as any man would do anything for his wife and children, I vowed to do anything and everything to stay with Keri and the kids. I popped another piece of biotin gum in my mouth to sooth the festering mouth sores, and then I held Keri's hand again.

By this time, I'd had three rounds of chemo. The effects on my body were evident, and I hoped the chemo was working to annihilate the cancer, which I regarded as my opponent. I postured, both mentally and physically, to steel myself for the battle ahead. Through the chemo and its endless side effects, I felt comfortable about one thing: *my job*. Not only did I need my job, but I also needed my health insurance if I was to continue the fight. For this reason, I continued to do my job, no matter how sick I felt or how weak I became.

"What can I get you?" Keri asked one morning as I sat at the bar in the kitchen, dressed for work but exhausted.

"Nothing. I'm just trying to get the energy to get in the car."

I'd gotten to the point where I knew what to expect and how to pace myself to find every ounce of energy throughout my day. If I got dressed then made it to the kitchen, I knew I could sit down and regroup for ten minutes so I could get into my car. Even the simplest, most mundane tasks became exhausting and draining.

"Go! Go! Go!" I mentally willed myself again and again when I didn't think I could take another step.

As I trudged into work, those words filled my head—even as I counted down the remaining steps into office. I half-smiled at people on the way in, careful not to waste energy with conversation or break my stride.

"Go! Go! Go!" I silently repeated until I finally got to my desk and sat down to catch my breath as I read the morning's e-mails and messages.

I hated the fact that I felt so weak. I resented that my body had betrayed me.

Where is the old Rob? I often wondered. *Where is the guy who could run for miles? Where is the guy who competed in triathlons and who always felt great? Will I ever see him again, or is he gone for good?*

The guy who I met at the mirror each morning looked gaunt,

with hollow eyes and dull, pale skin. He'd lost all his hair and even his eyebrows and eyelashes. He looked skinny and sick, more like a shell of a man than the guy I'd known my whole life.

"You're always handsome to me," Keri reminded me as she hugged me from the back as I looked in the mirror. "And I love you."

Her positive attitude and constant affirmations got me through some of my toughest days. She was beside me every step of the way. I'd always loved her, but when we faced down cancer together, we became even closer. On those days when I couldn't find the strength, she gave me hers until I could gather my own again. I think we both began to understand the true meaning of marriage. My "cute Keri" was even stronger than I'd thought.

Chemo four was on August 6. By that time, I knew what to expect and how to pace myself for what would happen. Keri was with me, as always, when the poison dripped into my veins, ready to do battle with the cancer and to stand with me as we defeated our enemy. She and I talked and joked, and as always, I was constantly amazed by her strength.

Keri's positive attitude became my rock and helped me to stay strong, even in the face of uncertainty. We both knew of all the possible sides effects and that many cancer patients experienced anxiety and depression during and after chemo treatments. With Keri by my side, it was easier to ward off at least *that* side effect.

After chemo four, I paced myself and waited a couple of days for the exhaustion, mouth sores, lack of appetite, and nausea to hit. It had become a predictable cycle by that time, and I knew what to expect, just as sure as I knew the sun would rise each morning.

When it became apparent that I simply couldn't eat though, Keri insisted we get to the hospital. I told her, "It'll pass. It always does. I can get through it."

Keri kept in constant touch with the chemo nurse. And she dealt with each side effect as it came, one at a time or several at a time.

I went to the office during this bout of side effects. As I talked with vendors and employees on the phone, I swallowed down the rising nausea as I fought to focus on our conversations. I felt cold constantly, and I couldn't stop my body from shivering. Between calls, reports, and e-mails, I went into the bathroom to put cold water on my face, though it never helped.

It got to the point that I could eat only soft breakfast foods. Keri made me lots of pancakes and eggs, and I ate many gummy bears.

By August 15, both Keri and I were surprised that the side effects hadn't relented at all. I grew weaker by the hour as I tried to plow through my work, but I was determined not to miss a beat and to keep up with my responsibilities. I was also running a low-grade fever. My doctor advised me not to worry about it and to alert him if it spiked.

It was then that I began to *really* feel the effects of what was happening inside my body. Since I was so weak, Keri let our friends and family know what was going on:

> Although Rob's been handling this like a champ, he's dealing with some side effects from the chemo, namely fatigue, mouth sores, and thrush. He has no appetite and finds it difficult to eat or talk because of the painful mouth sores. He says he feels "funky"—his words, not mine. He's spending time on his computer and trying to keep up with his work and I wish he'd rest more, but then we all know how he can be!

Not only did I feel sick, but I also knew Walter wanted me at work, even though I could barely hold my head up. Since I've always been a dependable person with a good work ethic, it bothered me that I was too sick to go to work. As a result, it was impossible to rest as my mind whirled and buzzed with all the responsibilities that called to me from the office.

In hindsight, I realize it would have been best for me to take a leave of absence from work, since I definitely would have qualified for it based on my circumstances. But I thought I could work through the chemo and just keep going as usual.

I really thought that if I could just rest and regain my strength, I'd get through it. Our yearly vacation to the Lake of the Ozarks was quickly approaching, and I wasn't sure how I'd find the energy to make the eleven-hour drive. "Listen, Keri," I said. "You and the boys just go on to the lake as planned. I'll be fine here."

"I'm not leaving you like this!" she insisted as she looked at me like I was crazy.

"No, the boys have been looking forward to going to the lake.

You all go ahead. Seriously, I'll be fine. You can't do anything for me here anyway. I'm just going to lie down and rest, so the peace and quiet here will be perfect for me."

Although it took some convincing, Keri relented and took the boys to meet my parents at Lake of the Ozarks for the regularly scheduled family trip. Since I had so little energy and felt totally drained, I went to bed and hoped I'd feel rested later. I slept fitfully, but I got up and went to work in the morning and then to a scheduled checkup with my doctor. My white blood cell count was drastically low.

"You need to remain isolated for rest of the week, Rob," the doctor advised. "I mean totally isolated—no work, no public places, not even tap water for you. You can drink only bottled water."

At the end of that visit, I felt even more exhausted, so I went home and went straight to bed. When I woke up hours later, I felt sicker, if that was even possible.

By the next day, I felt worse and worse. The thermometer confirmed my suspicions: 101.1. When I took my temperature again later, it was over 102.

Keri sent me a text: "How are you feeling?"

I sent her a photo of the thermometer beside me.

"That doesn't look good," she texted back.

"I'll be okay. I love you," I replied.

I learned later that Keri had caller her friend Dana and asked her to bring over cases of bottled water and some gummy bears because that was the only thing for which I had an appetite.

I went back to bed, pulled the covers up around my neck, and instantly fell asleep again. A little while later, I heard the doorbell ring at our side entrance. I was white as a ghost, and my breathing was shallow and labored as I opened the door.

"Wow! You look awful, Rob!" Dana said when she saw me. "Ker's worried about you, so I wanted to come by and check on you. I think we should go to the hospital."

Hours later, I was still in the hospital waiting room when Dana talked on the phone with Keri. "Rob looks really bad. He's pale and his breathing is shallow. It's scary. I'll stay with him until he's admitted. You should take the next flight home. I'll call you again in a few hours."

After several tests, the doctor came in to talk to me. "You have neutropenia due to the chemo," the doctor confirmed. "When you become neutropenic, your white blood count is abnormally low, and you're more susceptible to bacterial infections as a result. It's hard for the body to fight off infection. It can become life threatening, depending upon the duration. You've also got pneumonia, and that's why you're having difficulty breathing. It's a good thing you got to the hospital. We'll need to keep you isolated for a few days and get some IV antibiotics going. And we'll try to figure out what's causing the infection."

Keri took the next flight home and her friends Dana and Jill picked her up at the airport at one in the morning and brought her to the hospital. My parents stayed at the lake with the boys so Keri could be with me.

"I need to use your laptop," I told her minutes after she'd arrived.

"For what? You're supposed to be resting."

"I've got to let them know at work what's going on."

Keri brought me my laptop, and I opened one from my boss. "I've got a meeting in a couple days," I told Keri as she sat beside my hospital bed.

"You can hardly stand up!"

"Maybe I'll be better by tomorrow."

When my boss read the e-mail I'd sent him, he replied, "I'm here for you, Rob! Let me know if there's anything you need."

The doctors kept me in the hospital for three days and then sent me home.

"Bed rest, Rob. That's what you need," the doctor reminded me as he signed the release form. "We're not going to do the fifth or sixth chemo. Our goal is not to kill you! Go home and rest."

Keri shot me a knowing glance and shook her head.

After my three days in the hospital, I thought I felt good enough to go home. After a few more days, I even had a little bit of strength back. Keri wanted me to take more time to rest and to get stronger, but I felt I needed to get back to work. We later learned that an abscessed tooth had caused the infection that had sent me to the hospital.

"How can you go into work, Rob?" Keri asked one morning.

"You're exhausted after just getting dressed. You can barely even stand up."

"I'll be okay. Really."

A few hours later, Keri called me at work to see how I was doing. "Fine," I said. "But I'm freezing. I just can't get warm, no matter what I do."

An hour later, Keri showed up at my office with a sweater for me. "You need to be at home and in bed," she said as she kissed me goodbye. I put on the sweater.

"I'll see you tonight. Kiss the boys for me," I told her.

Although I felt worse than I'd ever felt in my life, I knew I needed to pull my weight at work. Since I had cancer, I was certain that I couldn't lose my job. My family was counting on me, and I had to keep my health insurance if I planned to continue treatment.

The next morning, I woke up and paced myself as I dressed, rested at the bar in our kitchen, and got in my car. Keri walked me outside and kissed me goodbye, but the look on her face told me she didn't approve of me going to work so soon.

I made it through the day and then the next one too, but on August 27, I called my boss to tell him I'd be working from home that day because I was still sick. The next day, I did the same thing. I'd been out of the office a twenty-three days between May and August.

The next morning, after I talked to human resources, I sent an e-mail to document our conversation for Hydeswort and I copied my boss, as always:

> Rick—
>
> Attached is the link to the Cancer calendar, along with the detail below. Access is available for this calendar to you, Walter and Scott. Anne also had access while she was still here. The calendar is kept up-to-date with all appointments, days off and information.
>
> In addition, I attached the "days off" spreadsheet that we reviewed today.
>
> Thanks for your time, and as always I will keep you up to speed on any changes.
>
> Rob Atteberry

7
The Way We Get By

By Spoon

In addition to the long list of unpleasant side effects from the chemo, I also had some teeth issues, another result of the chemo's assault on my body. I'd always dealt with teeth problems, but the chemo had further weakened my teeth and gums, which eventually led to a root canal and another crown, as if I needed even one more thing to deal with. I took it in stride though and went through each day one at a time.

The month of September went by, and my body slowly began to heal from the chemo that had invaded it in an effort to kill off the bad cancer cells. I *thought* things were progressing just as they should, and I worked my way through the exhaustion, the hair loss, and the fact that no foods tasted good anymore. I tried to take it all in stride.

On October 1, I kissed Keri goodbye and headed off to the office as I'd done countless times. My mind was on all the items on that day's calendar. I made mental notes of people I needed to call and things I needed to do while I headed to my new office, where Walter had recently relocated me.

Minutes later, seated at my desk, and as I looked at a report on my computer screen, my intercom buzzed. "Rob, I need to talk to you," Walter said.

"Sure. Be right there."

Thirty minutes later, I was in my car again, driving home in the early-morning sun. I felt like I'd been hit head-on by a train that I hadn't seen coming.

"Hey!" Keri said cheerfully as she answered my phone call.

"I'm on my way home," I said, feeling bruised and shell-shocked.

"Now? Why? Do you feel okay, Rob?" she panicked.

"They let me go, Keri. Walter just fired me. I'll see you in a few minutes and tell you about it."

As I pulled into our neat, manicured neighborhood, the grass was still wet with the morning dew. A woman walked behind a baby stroller, and another woman jogged along the street with earphones in her ears. It dawned on me that their worlds were calm, predictable, and peaceful, while my own had imploded with no warning.

I parked in our driveway and stoically went inside.

"What?" Keri asked as she dried her hands with a dishtowel and came over to me. "Why? I don't under—"

I walked into my home office, and Keri followed me.

I explained, still trying to digest it all myself. "Walter and Rick said my area is being reorganized, so they had to let two people go. Jim and I were it. Some other employees are being merged with another department."

"I can't believe it! You've been killing yourself for that company, even since you got sick," Keri said as she hugged me where I numbly sat at my desk, surrounded by shelves of thousands of neatly organized CDs.

"I don't get it either."

"Wait a minute, Rob. This is crazy. How can they let you go? I mean right *now*, just as you're going through cancer treatment?"

"I know. I'll have to cancel the radiation treatments that are scheduled to start October 20."

"You can't do that!"

"I won't have insurance though, Keri."

"We'll find a way."

"I just need to work it all out. I know we'll get by. I just don't want to tap into our savings, especially if I don't have a job."

"What did you say to them when they told you, Rob?"

"I said, 'I'll be talking to you,' and then I got up and left. My legs felt like lead weights as I walked out of there."

The rest of that first day of October was a blur as I played the bizarre scene over and over in my mind and tried to make sense of what had happened to upend my world. Cancer had come into my life abruptly and with no warning, and so had being let go from my job with no notice and at the worst possible time.

My stomach was twisted with anger, resentment, and absolute shock that Bruce, my onetime friend, had sanctioned my firing at all, much less when I was fighting for my life and battling cancer. He had brought me up in the ranks with Gechsmin, and then he'd asked me to come to Hydeswort and to work under Walter. The whole thing made no sense to me, and I felt like I'd been kicked in the stomach.

We had hit rock bottom, and as the husband and father, it was up to me to take control and fix things for us. I'd have given anything to have the energy to work on my newest problem, but I was having difficulty just wrapping my head around what had happened to me. I felt like I'd been sucker-punched, and I couldn't catch my breath.

My emotions ran the gamut. One minute I was furious, and the next I was worried. I'd done what was expected of me. I'd been a reliable, productive employee for Hydeswort, just like I'd been in any other position I'd ever held. It was in my makeup to be dependable and responsible, and I'd really presumed that if I held up my end of the employment deal, my employer would do the same. *Isn't that how it's supposed to be?*

We had money in the bank, but I knew radiation would be expensive. In addition to all the financial considerations, I was left with many questions about why my job had been summarily stripped from me like a defender strips a football from a ball carrier. But I wasn't in a football game, and I certainly didn't have the bank account of a professional athlete. I was but a typical, run-of-the-mill middle-class guy who presumed his employer would return his loyalty and humanity, especially at the worst time of his life.

Nonstop questions plagued me, although most of them were rhetorical, so they'd never be answered:

> *Did Walter see me as a threat, especially since he'd already had so many jobs over the span of his own career?*

> *Was he already trying to find a way to get rid of me when he moved me into a smaller, unimportant office across the hall?*

> *Why had I been given the boring, innocuous project when I'd successfully handled high-profile projects?*

> *Was I already sick with cancer when I went to Hydeswort?*

> *Did I have cancer when I was with Tendlart?*

> *Will I ever get any answers?*

I'd be lying if I said I wasn't somewhat frightened about how to proceed. I had worked so hard for so many years to get our family to a certain standard of living. Keri and I were proud of the spacious home we'd built for our boys and proud that we could give them the lives they deserved. I had been sure the cancer was just a stumbling block that I'd overcome. But I'd never expected to be unemployed, since I thought I'd done everything right. I'd come to work, even when I was so sick; I'd worked from home to pull my weight for the company; I'd made myself available day and night, no matter what, and I'd been a team player from day one.

"Mom and Dad think I should go on long-term disability," I told Keri.

"Well, I'm also getting a job," she proclaimed. "I'm going back to teaching."

"No, not yet. I'll figure it out."

"I was going to go back to teaching anyway," she insisted. "And the twins are older, so it's time."

"Okay, I'll look into long-term disability while you see about a teaching job."

We'd always been a team, but this time it felt different. I wasn't leading the team like I'd always done, and she was shouldering more of the burden than I was comfortable with. To make matters worse, we had no playbook.

"We'll get through this," Keri said as she hugged me. "You'll see."

While I contemplated things, Keri sent an e-mail to her best girlfriends:

Hi Girls,

Sorry I've been hard to reach for a couple days. Things are insane right now. Rob and I are still trying to digest what's happened. I really just don't get it. He gave his all to his job—even when he was so sick that he could barely even stand. On the days when I begged him not to go in to the office, he said he "had a responsibility to the company" and that he'd "be fine." What kind of people would fire a guy who's dealing with cancer? It seems heartless, at the very least. Rob seems lost right now. He's always worked so hard and he was proud of how far he's come and at such a young age. It's like they pulled the rug out from under him at the very worst time of him life, and with no warning at all. I just can't believe this happened. I'm sure we'll be okay, we just need to take some time and figure out what to do. Anyway, thanks for letting me vent. Gotta run.

Keri

I delayed my upcoming radiation appointments and consulted an attorney. He told me that nine out of ten times, a sick employee's employer puts him on long-term disability in similar situations. But when I talked to Hydeswort, I was told disability wasn't a possibility for me, since I'd already been removed from the company and severed as an employee.

So, I was fired less than twenty-four hours ago, and they've got no record that I even worked there? I was furious.

I felt overwhelmed and abandoned, like a fish floundering on a dock and gasping for breath. So much of my identity and how I viewed myself in the world was tied up in my corporate identity. My new world seemed dark, uncertain, and foreboding as I planned my next steps.

Keri, who is usually calm and even-tempered, was angry with the company and continued to worry about my health. "What they did to you is wrong. It's just plain *morally wrong*. But the priority right now is for you to start radiation. We need to get you well."

While I dealt with my health and the impending disaster brought on by my employer, Keri maintained our family and our home life. Meanwhile, my attorney contacted Hydeswort about our intent to sue for wrongful termination. I found it odd that Bruce and Walter denied having known that I had cancer.

"Not only did they know," I told my attorney, "but Walter and I exchanged e-mails on it. I'll give you copies of the correspondence."

Because I was so grateful to be done with chemo and I just wanted to get on with my life, I moved on to the next stage of my battle and began radiation treatments. At least I had the insurance concerns handled.

Radiation treatments turned out to be an intense experience. On the first day, I lay still on a table while several technicians fitted a soft piece of plastic around my head and molded an exact replica of my head and face. *This whole process is so bizarre,* I thought. *How did I get to this point?*

At least a thousand times in the many months prior, I'd

wondered how I could possibly be dealing with cancer and all it entailed. It just didn't seem possible that I'd gone through all I had and was still ensnared in cancer's grasp. But I was determined to fight each battle and to *win* the war.

The radiation treatments required that I go to my doctor's office at the same time each day for twenty-one straight days. The entire process, from the minute I arrived, took twenty minutes, with the actual radiation lasting less than five minutes. The radiologist decided to administer the lowest possible dosage, since the targeted area was so close to my brain.

Each day, I lay still on a cold, hard table in a still, sterile room with the specially made plastic mask fitted over my head. Without moving, my eyes watched as the gigantic machine navigated slowly around my head.

Stay positive! I silently reminded myself as I thought of Keri and the boys. *You've got this! You'll beat it! Go! Go! Go!*

I willed myself to stay positive and hopeful, although I was overwhelmed. Yet it gave me comfort to know that Keri waited faithfully in the other room for my treatment to finish and that I'd again see her reassuring smile in just a couple of minutes. She had a strength within her that was both a blessing and a powerful source of strength to me.

I thought often of the wedding vow that reminds us we promise to be there for our partner "in sickness and in health." When I married Keri, I never could have imagined there would come a time when *I* would need to lean on *her*. But she was there for me, steadfast and strong, when I needed her most.

On the days when Keri was busy with the kids, my dad took

me to radiation treatments. With him there, I felt a different kind of strength, a different sort of empowerment and encouragement that was almost tangible. It was as if Dad willed his strength and positivity to me when I needed it most, yet no words were needed between father and son.

Boys look up to their fathers as their first heroes, often trying to emulate and imitate their strength and character. While I may have been a grown man and a father, Dad would never know how much it meant to have him there with me.

Since we'd never before been through radiation, none of us had any idea what a big event it was when a patient completed his final treatment. We later learned about the traditional bell-ringing ceremony that signified it. Unaware of the coming celebration, I drove myself to my last treatment.

Immediately after my last radiation, the kind nurses walked me back to the waiting room and cheered and clapped as I rang the bell that marked my final treatment. I felt hopeful as I drove away.

When I got home later that day, Keri had a big bunch of balloons and a candy-bar bouquet waiting for me. I was amazed that she was so thoughtful in the wake of all she'd been going through, but then again, that's Keri, the nicest person I've ever met!

After radiation, I had scans done to see whether the chemo and the radiation had worked. The word *remission* had never had more meaning or sounded so good.

8
A Pain That I'm Used To

By Depeche Mode

 New Year's 2013 brought with it the hope and promise of a brighter future like no year before it. Keri and I felt we'd battled the cancer beast and had won. Unbeknownst to me at the time, Keri was still worried. She texted a friend.

> I can't put my finger on it, but Rob seems a little out of it sometimes. Maybe it's a bit of depression, which I know affects some people when they fight cancer. I just miss his smile and his sense of humor around the house.

Though I was officially declared in remission by February, Keri still bore the brunt of caring for our four boys. She and I presumed I was still fatigued because of all I'd been through in the last few months.

We wanted to bring some fun and laughter back into the house, so we got a puppy for the boys in February. Like all puppies, ours had the occasional accident while being housebroken. But my lackluster response to the puppy's accident one day was out of the ordinary.

Keri came into the family room and asked, "Rob, what's wrong with you?"

"What do you mean?" I asked in a monotone voice.

"The puppy, Rob! The puppy threw up on the floor, and the boys are running all around, and you're not even paying attention to any of it!" she said. "What's going on?"

I heard her voice, but neither her words nor her exasperation registered with me. The house could have been on fire, for all I knew, and I had literally *no reaction* to anything or anyone. I was physically there, but mentally and cognitively I felt trapped inside my physical form, unable to participate in life.

The old Rob would have sprung into action, cleaned up the puppy's mess, reprimanded him, and taken control of the boys as they ran around the house. The new Rob couldn't seem to connect the dots to respond to anything; he merely observed life as a silent spectator.

Keri texted my sister, Cindy:

> It's like he has no reaction—to anything! He sits and stares at the TV, but he's not really watching it. It's as if he's here, but he's NOT here. He sleeps constantly! He doesn't even smile anymore! It's like he's tuned out and shut off from everything! Something's very wrong! I'm really worried.

As I slept away my days or sat stoically and unaffected, Keri cared for the boys and handled our family's needs. In addition to all that, she gave me my medications, prepared food for me when I felt like eating, and helped me to do everything—and I mean *everything*. She bathed the boys and tucked them into their beds each night then helped me walk upstairs, helped me take a shower, and tucked me into bed, too. Basically, she had five Atteberry boys, but one of us was old enough to vote.

She soon insisted that I see a doctor to find out what was wrong with me. I'm sure her heart was broken, since she'd basically lost her husband, but she tried to stay focused, even with all the stress and responsibilities she carried at the time.

"It's PTSD," the doctor diagnosed. "It happens sometimes after people go through cancer treatment. Plus, he lost his job, and that was a big part of his identity and how he related to the world and his place in it. We can prescribe some antidepressants. I'd also like to send him for a sleep study to see if he's getting adequate oxygen while sleeping. If he's not, that explains why he's so tired. We'll take care of him. He'll be fine."

The doctor also suggested I see a therapist to talk about how I'd been feeling. Keri had a friend from high school who was a therapist specializing in treating cancer patients, so she made me an appointment.

Keri texted this to my sister:

I've started keeping notes about what Rob is doing. It's weird, almost like he's looking thru me, not AT me. It's like he's physically here, but not really

HERE. He'll be with your parents at the lake soon.

Let's see what they think.

Keri continued to try and engage me in conversation and to get some sort of response from me, other than a bland one-word reply. One day I was driving and pulled into our subdivision then just stopped in the middle of the entrance for no obvious reason.

"Rob, are you going to keep driving?" Keri asked from the passenger seat.

"Uh, oh, yeah," I replied.

Because of that episode, coupled with other things she'd noticed, she took over the driving.

Even I realized I'd ceased communicating with people, although I couldn't articulate my concerns. When I did speak, it was an effort. Even then, Keri could hear me only if she leaned in and put her ear next to my mouth. "I'm sorry I'm not talking much," I said a few times. "I don't know why."

The sleep study revealed nothing. My oxygen levels were adequate when I slept, so that wasn't the source of the problem.

"Oh, he'll snap out of it," the doctor told Keri when she talked to him. "Give the medication time to work. It has to build up in Rob's system, and it's got a residual effect that multiplies over time. I'm sure he'll be just fine. You've both been through a lot in the last year. Give it some time."

Keri grew more and more concerned with each passing day. She talked with her friends and our family and e-mailed everyone about what had been happening:

Hi All,

Sorry for the blanket mass email. It's been another long day and I just got the kids to bed, so it's late. Things aren't getting any better; in fact, Rob seems worse. It's definitely more than depression. We were outside today in the yard, and he lost his balance and fell over again for the third time. He was just standing there and he toppled over. That's *not* depression. It seems like the doctors are completely missing it and I'm getting more worried. Thanks for checking in on him. I'll let you know if we learn anything new.

Keri

When I went to the lake to stay with my parents in May, it gave Keri a welcome break. I didn't know it, but she had talked with them and asked them to observe me and make notes, just as she'd done.

"I see what you mean," my mom told Keri. "He's not talking as much, he's walking funny, and one of his shoulders is drooped. I've looked up the symptoms on the Internet, and it really seems like it might be a stroke."

"Possibly," Keri replied. "I just don't know, Diane. He's not himself—not at all. I really miss the old Rob. I'll go with him to his next appointment with the therapist, and I'll tell her what we've talked about."

Our family jokingly refers to my mom as Dr. Atteberry because she constantly researches symptoms and tries to diagnose family members with her WebMD findings. It's one of the things we love about Mom; she would go to the ends of the earth for her kids. Research was Mom's way of doing all she could to help Keri and me.

When it was time for my next appointment with the therapist, Keri accompanied me. I sat quietly and emotionless as the two of them discussed my behavior. I watched their mouths move, and I heard their voices, but what they said didn't register at all. I was a mute, contented onlooker while the two women talked about me. Still undiagnosed, I was basically trapped inside a failing, diminishing shell, and time wasn't on my side.

"Look, Keri," the therapist said. "I've been reading about PSTD, and Rob *doesn't* have the symptoms of PTSD. I think it's something physical that's going on with him."

"We're supposed to go on a family trip next week," Keri told her. "It's a Disney cruise with the whole family. Should we still go?"

"I think you can take him. They'll have a doctor on the ship. But keep an eye on him, and don't leave him alone until we can figure this thing out."

Our family of six, my parents, my sister, her husband, and their kids all went to Florida to set sail on the Disney cruise. I was very quiet and entirely exhausted, even from the moment we set foot on the cruise ship. The boys danced around and enjoyed the bon voyage party on deck as the ship pulled out of port. Just watching them made me tired, but I presumed my body hadn't bounced back from all I'd be through. I didn't have the energy to make conversation or the desire to engage with people.

After breakfast the next day, I sat at the pool with my family but was too exhausted to do anything else. I went back to our cabin for a nap, and I was asleep in no time.

"Hey," Keri said as she rubbed my back, "wake up, Rob. It's time for dinner."

"Dinner?" I asked. "How long was I sleeping?"

"Since one. It's after six now. Are you hungry?"

"A little."

"Well, we're going to meet everyone in the dining room in thirty minutes."

Even a shower didn't energize me, and I was more fatigued than ever after I dressed for dinner. Keri took my hand, led me from our cabin and into the hall, and then guided me toward the elevators. I quietly walked beside her and was glad she was leading the way. I'd learn later that it broke her heart to take my hand, as if I were one of our boys, but in front of me she was nothing but loving and strong.

The boys happily entertained each other during dinner, but the adults around our table seemed quieter than usual as they looked at me and then glanced at one another. I was too exhausted to ask what was going on, and I didn't really care at the time. Dinner seemed to take too long, and I was relieved when the waiter removed all the dessert and coffee dishes. I could barely hold my eyes open, and I told Keri I needed to go to bed.

"I'll walk back to the room with you," she said as she took my hand. "And then I'll come back and join the others on the deck."

"We'll take the boys over to the Kids' Club," Diane offered. "You two go ahead."

When I was back in bed again, Keri tucked me in and then went to find our family on the upper deck. They were all seated around a table and having drinks under the stars.

"The boys are at the Kids' Club," my mom told Keri. "We'll go back for them in a little while."

"Okay, thanks." Keri sipped the drink they'd ordered for her, and then she said sadly, "He's getting worse."

"We can tell," my sister, Cindy, agreed. "We've all been talking about it."

"I'm so worried," Keri said. "Something's just not right. This isn't depression. It's not PTSD. *What's* going on with him? He just keeps saying he's tired, but that's not it either. He's got an appointment with his oncologist on the day after we get back. Hopefully we can get some answers."

The next morning, we got off the ship and went ashore for an excursion. I followed our group, uncertain of where we were going and not sure I cared. It was as if I were on autopilot as my legs moved in sync with theirs—left, right, left, right. I stopped when my family did, and then I silently resumed my robotic pace alongside them.

Back on the ship, I took a nap again and awoke to find Keri curled up in a chair and writing in her journal. "Hey, whatcha doing?" I asked.

"Just writing about our day so I don't forget anything."

"Okay, I'm going to sleep a little longer."

Keri went back to her writing as the sun set outside.

> What is going on with Rob? I handed our passports to him, so he could hand them to the guy as we got back on the ship, but he's so robotic, like he's not really here and engaging with people. His dad had to help him and guide him all day, saying, "Walk here, Rob; turn here; sit here" all day. I'm terrified that the old Rob is gone, but I'm even more scared that something awful is happening and the doctors haven't identified it. This was not the vacation I'd imagined—not at all.

While I slept, Keri went to my parents' cabin and found Cindy and her husband there. Everyone looked concerned, and it was clear they'd all been talking about me.

"It's like his sense of humor is completely gone," Keri agreed. "He doesn't engage with anyone like he used to—not even the boys."

My mom and my sister fought back tears.

"It's like—like he's a zombie," Keri added. "I even miss arguing with him. I miss his type-A personality and how he'd freak out over the smallest things."

My dad hugged her and said, "Well, let's make the best of it, and we'll talk to the doctors when we get home again."

Everyone continued to accommodate me during our family trip. Because I was always so tired, they had to leave activities early to get me back to my cabin so I could take naps. We'd even eat dinner earlier than usual, so I could get to bed. Thankfully, we had family with us, because I was unable to interact with our boys myself.

After a few more days at sea, our family was back in Florida and at Universal Studios in Orlando. Keri videotaped us as we walked around and went on the various rides throughout the day. My legs felt like lead, and I stumbled at times as I tried to keep pace with everyone while keeping my balance. The boys had a good time as our family enjoyed the Florida sunshine.

I'M
DONE !
11/12/12

Rob Atteberry's Survivor Story

SUR VI VOR

ancer Cente

Kicking Cancer's A**

9
Everything Is Wrong

By Interpol

B ack at home again, several days later, Keri told my mom she had been taking video on our trip to show to my oncologist.

"Here," my mom said, "take this letter too. I'm Rob's mother, and I've known him all his life. A mother always knows when something's not right with her children. The doctor may have his MD, but I've got my MOM and many more years of experience in knowing my son. I want that doctor to hear from me while he views Rob on the videotape you're taking to him."

Keri and I visited my oncologist, and she immediately insisted he view the videotape and read my mom's detailed letter of the changes she saw in me. I'd never seen Keri be so forceful, pushy, insistent. She'd always been the polite, nice, mannerly one.

The doctor viewed the video that showed me trying to keep my balance as my shoulder drooped and I stumbled a few times while I shuffled along. "I see what you mean," the doctor said.

"Our therapist said she doesn't believe he has PTSD," Keri explained as she pushed the therapist's report toward the doctor.

"Has he had an MRI done of his brain?"

"No," Keri replied. "Just a PET scan."

"Well, that wouldn't show his brain," the doctor said.

"What?! I thought PET scans also show what's happening in the brain. Why have we not checked his brain?"

"We will now. I will schedule an appointment immediately."

I observed their exchange as if silently watching a tennis match from the sideline. I heard their voices volley back and forth, and yet their comments weren't entirely registering with me. But I trusted that Keri would handle things, and in a few minutes I followed her out of the office and back to our car.

"You're going to have an MRI, Rob," Keri explained. "Maybe we'll get some answers."

Two days later, the MRI was done in the morning. Hours later, Keri and I were in the car as she was driving our boys home from a trampoline center in town. With the boys buckled in back, she drove along as her cell phone rang.

"Are you driving?" the doctor asked her.

"Yes," I heard her answer into the phone.

"Well, pull over if you can, Keri."

I watched as Keri pulled our Suburban off the road, put it in park, pulled a pad and pen out of the console under her right elbow, and then got out. She was in front of the car with the phone to her ear, writing on the pad and leaning on the car's hood as cars whizzed by. I couldn't hear what she said, but she looked concerned, and her eyes looked sad.

A couple of minutes later, Keri opened the driver's door and got behind the wheel again. The pad was in a cup holder between the front seats. I watched her and knew she was anxious as she pulled the Suburban back onto the road again. She was oddly calm, and she didn't offer any information.

"What is it?" I finally asked.

She swallowed hard as she glanced in the rearview mirror. Then she began to speak as the boys happily chattered in the backseats. "The doctor said the MRI showed an abnormality. He wants to do an MRI spectroscopy to have a closer look at your brain tissue. It's a better MRI that'll show definitive details and indicate whether it's *specifically* lymphoma. The doctor said the scan lights up like a Christmas tree if lymphoma is present. The abnormality might be nothing at all or it might—" Keri paused. "Or it might—or it might be lymphoma."

I watched as she swallowed hard and focused at the road ahead. I knew her well enough to know she fought back tears because the boys were in the car with us. They didn't know about all we'd been going through, and we'd wanted to spare them the worries we'd had. Children shouldn't have to know about awful things like cancer. Their childhood innocence shouldn't be touched by such dreadful realities.

The boys happily talked in the back, aggravating each other as boys do, and joked around while music played from the car's speakers. Keri touched her left cheek as she cleared her throat and then reached for my hand as she quietly drove on.

I'd look back on that time and realize just how strong my wife had been that day. But in that moment I was in a fog-like stupor, so I couldn't relate to her emotions.

Later that evening, the boys were playing and I was asleep, as usual. Keri got a call from my doctor to check in with her and finalize the details of the MRI spectroscopy, scheduled for the next day. As she answered her phone, she rushed outside and onto our front porch to find a quiet place where she could talk with the doctor. The boys had been used to being quiet while I was on a business call, but this was entirely different. Besides, it had been months since I'd had been on a business call, so the boys weren't used to having to keep it down during a phone conversation.

"*Now* do you believe me, Doctor?" Keri asked after briefly listening. "I've been trying to tell you something's very wrong!"

"I do. Yes, I do. He definitely has a brain abnormality."

The doctor went on tell Keri the time of my scan, and they went over a few more details. By this time, Keri felt qualified to have medical conversations with my doctors, based on what I'd been through and all she'd learned about cancer, treatments, side effects, and even mortality rates. It was nothing she'd ever wanted to know and nothing she'd expected to ever touch her family, but these things had become a real part of our world. Keri steeled herself and continued the conversation.

I had the MRI spectroscopy, and we waited for the results. While I slept enough for a half-dozen people, Keri could barely sleep at all. She continued to go through the motions of handling the boys and our family routines.

Every time her phone rang, Keri grabbed it, eager to hear the results. Her heart pounded like a jackhammer in her chest when the next day she recognized the doctor's phone number on her phone's screen. She walked outside as she answered the call.

Not even a minute later, the color had drained from her face as she held her stomach and shut her eyes. The doctor continued speaking as she tried to remain calm and just breathe.

"Okay, Doctor, so what's the plan?" she asked. "If the lymphoma is back, then what's our plan?"

"First, we'll need to drill a small hole in his head and do a biopsy to confirm that it's lymphoma."

"But you think it is," Keri said.

"Most likely, yes. And if it is lymphoma, we'll do intense chemotherapy with bone-marrow shots and a stem-cell transplant," he answered. "But it'll be an intense schedule. Rob will have four rounds of chemo in the hospital over a three-week period each time. Then he'll be home for a two-week break between rounds. It'll be tough and very regimented."

Keri walked down our driveway as she contemplated what I was in for and how she'd tell me. By this point, I barely spoke at all, and if I did, my voice was only a weak, hoarse whisper. Keri had to lean over and put her ear by my mouth to hear me.

She mulled over the doctor's plan for me and summoned her courage to ask the biggest question, for which she wasn't sure she wanted an answer: "Doctor, is it—is it *worth* it? I mean, is it worth putting him through all that?"

For Keri, it felt like I'd already been gone for months. The real Rob, the man she'd married, hadn't been in our home for so long. Her partner and the father of her children had disappeared and had left a hollow shell that resembled her husband only physically. Keri hadn't heard my laugh, shared jokes with me, or felt like her husband was with her for a long time. To her, it was as if I'd already gone away and left her, and she'd been mourning her lost husband for the last five months as she had stoically pushed onward with the demands of life.

"Oh, Keri," the doctor sighed. "I know what you're asking."

"Look, I've done all the research, Doctor. I know what he's up against. Please just level with me!" she begged. "What are his chances for recovery—for a *full* recovery?"

By this point, Keri felt the doctor was also a friend. She was sure he knew what she was going through, that he empathized with her, and that she could trust him.

"Well, *if* the treatment works—*if* it works—he'll have one year, maybe two—*if* he's lucky."

Never before had that little two-letter word meant so much. Not in all her years had Keri placed so much hope in the conjunction *if* as she thought of our boys and our family. She finally broke down and sobbed, and so did the doctor.

Keri tried to digest what she'd heard. "I've known Rob since I was eight years old! What do I do?"

She paced in our driveway and choked on her sobs as she tried to figure out what to do next. While she and I had always discussed things and made big decisions together, Keri was alone. She weighed the options and considered what my quality of life might be and for what period of time.

Keri wanted to make the right decision for me, since I couldn't make it for myself. She didn't want to put me through the treatment for *her*, for the boys, or for purely selfish reasons. It had to be the best decision for me, as an individual. Keri tried to separate her decision from her emotions, rationally considering the options and just thinking clearly.

"Keri, listen to me," the doctor finally said. "Whether or not we treat this isn't an option. Rob's too young and too strong *not* to treat it."

The doctor's positivity and his affirmative declaration were just what Keri needed to hear. His words gave her renewed strength and helped her to refocus again. "I need to talk to Rob's family. I'm not sure what to do. I'm not sure what's right, but I want to do what Rob would want."

"How about if I meet with all of you, and we can discuss things?" he offered.

"Yes. Yes, thank you."

Keri hung up with the doctor and then walked toward our front yard and sat down in the grass to dial Cindy. She regurgitated all the things the doctor had told her, and then they both broke down and sobbed together. Not a lot of words were exchanged as they wept together. It was one of those times when words weren't needed.

When Cindy could speak again, she assured her, "We can all talk about it and help you with this."

Keri hung up and went inside again. The boys were still playing together, unaware of the monster that threatened to take away their father and the happy family life they'd always known. It broke Keri's heart to think of the boys without their father. She went upstairs and found me asleep, just as she'd expected. She climbed into bed next to me and put her head on my chest.

I cuddled her closer without opening my eyes as she began to speak in a soft, sad voice. "It's in your brain, Rob. Lymphoma is in your brain."

I opened my eyes and looked down into hers, which were wet with tears. "Okay," I said with no emotion, as if she'd just said something innocuous like I needed to change a light bulb or take out the trash. Yet what she'd said did register with me on some level. It meant I had something else to do and something else to worry about in my tired, foggy state.

"I need to get a job then," I said. "If something happens to me, I need to make sure you and the kids are okay." It was clear I hadn't gotten over being let go from Hydeswort. It had been a painful blow that had cut me to the core and made me question who I was as a man, a husband, and a father. When I was a busy executive, I'd been in control of my world, responsible to many people, and proud of my accomplishments. But when Hydeswort pulled the rug from under me, I'd been left shaken and rattled, and I was no longer sure of how or where I fit into the world. The question "Who am I?" often plagued me.

Keri and I lay together, quietly holding each other and contemplating our uncertain future. The sounds of our boys playing and laughing reminded me of my biggest worry: *What will happen to them and to Keri if I'm not around for them?* It was all so unfair—not just to me, but to all of us. And I was too exhausted to deal with it, so I shut my eyes and fell asleep again.

10
Clinically Dead

By Chad Vangaalen

When I phoned my parents to tell them our latest bad news, Mom answered. She listened quietly as I shared what Keri had learned from my doctor. Mom had always been strong, in control, and not overly emotional, so I knew she got off the phone quickly so she could cry in private.

My parents and Keri's dad joined Keri and me at the University of Michigan to get a second opinion. Keri's mom watched the boys for us that day. As always, I followed our little entourage, matching their steps and taking a seat when they did.

While I was physically in the room, it was as if I weren't there as an integral part of what went on around me. I was merely a passive observer. Everyone discussed *me*, asked questions, and made the decisions for me as I watched and listened, unable to participate in the exchanges.

This was a whole new dynamic for our marriage, since I had always done the planning for our family. But on that day, Keri jumped in and shouldered the burden. I'd look back later and realize she'd always been capable of handling things, but I'd always felt the need to take care of things for our family.

The meeting that day yielded an option other than drilling into my brain. Dr. Junck, my doctor at the University of Michigan, had a different take on things. "Why drill?" he said. "There's a ninety-nine-point-nine percent likelihood that it's lymphoma. I think we need to skip the biopsy and just start treatment."

As Dr. Junck began the paperwork, and my mom brought out some papers she'd brought from home. "Doctor," she said, "this is some research I found online about a new way to treat lymphoma in the brain."

"Ahhhh, yes," Dr. Junck said as he looked at it. "I actually worked on this."

The research article discussed a special cocktail of chemotherapy and medications that are easier on the body but aggressively attack the cancer cells. The brain naturally protects itself, but Dr. Junck's methods allowed the medications to cross the natural barrier and get to the cancer cells.

He said, "Our plan will be to treat Rob over four or five days and then give him four to five weeks off, as opposed to Beaumont's plan that would put him in the hospital for three weeks at a time and then out for two."

The conversation continued, and it sounded intelligent and thoughtful. Everyone seemed to be working together to come up with a plan for me. Again, it was a bizarre scene, as I sat, a mute onlooker, while others discussed what would be best for me.

I heard all their words, and I saw how serious everyone's demeanor was, but I couldn't process the gravity of what they said.

It seemed like they were all a team though, all working toward the same goal. Then heads began to nod around me. In time, I silently filed out with my family, got in our car, and went home again, where I took a much-needed nap.

I knew Keri talked to our family and friends, but she also wrote her thoughts in a journal as a way of coping:

> Rob has been slowly leaving me, slipping away a bit at a time. How I wish he were here with me, juggling things and helping me to figure out what to do! It feels like I've been widowed for months now. He's physically here, right beside me; and yet I'm still so lonely without him.
>
> I guess this is what it's like to be a single parent. What's so hard though is the overwhelming sadness and loneliness. It breaks my heart to not have my partner here to talk with and laugh with.
>
> I'd do anything to have my husband back with me, but this time has also revealed a side of me that's given me a new sense of strength and independence too. Who knew I could repair things around the house? Who knew I could deal with our bills, budgeting, and running our entire household? Who knew I'd be our family's primary caretaker?

It would be so nice to hear Rob's laughter again though, or to see his eyes light up—or even to have an argument with him! I miss him. I'm grateful to stay so busy or else I know I'd be swallowed whole by the overwhelming sadness.

As one day melded into the next, I heard the words that swirled all around me, but my brain couldn't respond to what I heard. Sometimes I wanted to participate, but the words wouldn't come to my lips. They were locked away somewhere deep inside, and try as I might, I just couldn't bring them out.

It had been that way for six frustrating and exhausting months. I'd felt trapped inside my own body, just existing, but not engaging with others and not really living. It was a lonely place, just as Keri was also in her own lonely place, though I didn't know it then. We were right beside each other, yet we couldn't connect anymore. It was much more difficult for her because she understood what was happening and she still had to take care of our boys—and *me*.

During those days, I thought about what it might be like to die. I had questions, although I couldn't talk to anyone about them. They were buried deep inside my head, locked away and far from ever escaping my lips, because I couldn't form even simple sentences anymore.

The kids had gotten used to the fact that Dad slept all the time and Mom took care of them and ran the household. Dad was just *there*, breathing but emotionless, *existing* but not really *living*. Keri struggled with explaining the situation to them. When the cancer was in my sinuses, they knew "Daddy's nose is sick." Now Keri told them, "Daddy's brain is sick." I knew in my heart that I loved my wife and my children, but I could no longer express it to them. My heart knew it, but my brain wouldn't give me the words to tell them. I had no expression and no reaction to anything or anyone.

There was no joy, no laughter, no sadness, and no fear. There was nothing. It felt as if my emotions had been drained from my body. I felt hollow and empty, a shell without contents. Just the thought of trying to articulate my thoughts was exhausting.

My family realized the cancer had affected the parts of my brain that controlled my speech; all I knew was that I felt entirely disconnected from the world and everyone in it. It was as if the world moved on around me, but I couldn't keep up anymore. I couldn't engage with anyone or anything. I'd once been able to juggle a dozen things at once while also thinking about several more, but I couldn't grasp the simplest concepts anymore.

What is happening to me? I wondered inside my lonely shell.

Keri continued to field phone calls, e-mails, and texts from friends and family. She often resorted to texting to let people know what was going on.

> Thank you all for keeping in touch. We feel comfortable with Dr. Junck at U of M and so we're moving ahead. There are multiple spots in Rob's brain that are affected. They're not actually attached though. They're like "wisp" that freely "float" around in the center of Rob's brain, making

it impossible to go in and remove the cancer. We just hope and pray the treatment works. I'll keep you up-to-date on things. Thank you all for your continued prayers!

Keri and our families made the decision to move forward. Before starting treatment, Keri decided to throw a Kicking Cancer Again party. All of our close friends and family came over for Mexican food and margaritas. I sat at the kitchen counter, silently staring at the granite, while everyone I loved greeted me and wished me well. I barely reciprocated during conversations; I just ate the food Keri put in front of me and sat silently.

I vaguely remember this get-together. I've been told that a lot of people who came were startled to see my sallow face and blank eyes. E-mails and text updates didn't properly convey how serious the situation was. Many people left with tears in their eyes and continued crying on the drive home. The situation was grim, and now everyone knew it firsthand.

My loved ones were cautiously optimistic as my treatment began the next week. I was in the hospital for four days, but once again, I was never alone. Both Keri's parents and my parents rotated turns staying with our boys so Keri could be with me.

I think of my boys and then of my dad and the relationships I had with all of them. I imagine how hard it must have been for my father to watch what was happening to his son. Even in my altered state, I knew how terrifying it would be for me if one of our boys had cancer. But just like always, Dad was optimistic and positive on the outside, as was everyone in our family.

The treatments took about four hours, and as we waited, the chemo cocktail slowly dripping from the IV into my veins. It was strange to think about the medicine killing off the bad cancer cells, since it meant good cells would be destroyed too. But there didn't seem to be better options.

The process was very regimented and orderly, as each step was administered one at a time. The day before a treatment, I received sodium bicarbonate every four hours to protect my kidneys. On the first day of a three-hour chemo treatment, I also received antinausea meds and Benadryl. On the next day, I got cytarabine, a rough med that crossed the blood/brain barrier to kill cancer cells by interfering with DNA synthesis. All this was followed by a constant saline flushes to clear out toxins.

The doctors and nurses had their routines, and Keri and I also created ours. She and I passed the time watching TV shows like *Breaking Bad*. Keri lowered the AC thermostat in my room and brought our own blankets from home so we could be comfortable. On Tuesdays, we spent the entire day watching a *Law and Order: SVU* marathon. On Thursdays, the hospital cafeteria baked chocolate peanut-butter bars, and Keri and I always split one. Every day at three, she brought me a Starbucks frappuccino.

So we had a little routines we fell into, but no matter what, we kept our spirits high, and we laughed. We *always* laughed together, which reminds me of the saying "Laughter is the best medicine."

During my treatments, Keri also began online classes to renew her teaching certification. While I slept, she did her required reading—unless it was a Tuesday, when we watched *Law and Order: SVU*. We always joked that it was impossible for Keri to study on those days.

We tried to keep things as normal as possible. To that end, my parents sometimes brought the boys to visit me at the hospital. We'd all walk down the hallways together as they talked.

As Dr. Junck had explained, we did the chemo treatments in four-day intervals, went home for a few weeks, and then returned again for another IV cocktail, starting the process all over again. Since Keri and I had always loved movies, she and I made dates out of the repetitive process, going to a movie before my treatments started. The movies provided a welcome respite from all that was going on. For a couple of hours anyway, Keri and I could get away and feel normal again, even if only until the credits began to roll on the movie screen.

Keri's biggest fear was that the Rob she had known was gone forever and would never return to her. After the second round of chemo, she shared my progress in a text:

> He's coming back! It's like a light switch has been flipped and I've started to see the old Rob again! He smiled this morning and made a sarcastic comment about his breakfast. It was amazing!

During my treatments, I'd sometimes have a problem with urine incontinence, possibly a result of the lymphoma disrupting messages to my brain. At times I'd have no warning whatsoever, and Keri would leap up and help me race into the bathroom.

Occasionally, I didn't make it in time, so Keri started bringing spare clothes for me to the treatments. She soon learned where to find extra gowns and scrubs on that floor of the hospital too.

It was a good thing that my treatments were done at the hospital because the doctors were able to give me additional antinausea meds to combat the nausea waves that came with the chemo. The meds helped so much. I vomited only during my first round of treatment, when we didn't yet realize nausea was going to be a problem.

Keri stayed by my side and slept in a chair beside my bed; it reclined to become a makeshift bed. It couldn't have been comfortable, but she did it, And I was comforted with her beside me. When we were put in a private room, Keri could at least shower. But sometimes we shared a room with another patient, so that wasn't possible.

Our family and friends all pitched in to help us while Keri put all her energies into my treatments and communicating with my doctors. While I had hardly any strength, she seemed to have the strength of ten men. I marveled at all she did with a positive attitude and a ready smile.

If the number of people who love a man determines his true wealth, I must be the wealthiest man alive. The continuous messages of encouragement and nonstop prayers meant so much to me, and sometimes they came at just the right time. Some were simple texts, others were phone calls or notes, but there was a constant stream of love and support and messages like these:

Way to go, Rob! Kick cancer's butt!

Great news!

You're doing great! Get some rest!

We're praying for you, Rob! You've got this!

We didn't realize how many good friends and family members we had until this time. Besides all the calls, e-mails, and texts, people went out of their way to make our lives easier. My mom and my cousin Michele, along with two of Keri's friends, cleaned our entire house while Keri and I were away at the hospital. They even left fresh flowers for us.

Keri's mom made sure the kids' laundry was always washed and neatly put away. Keri's friends regularly took her out for "girl's nights" and checked in to make sure she was handling everything okay. They were her rock, and they proved that *family* doesn't only mean sharing the same bloodlines.

My friends pitched in too, especially when they thought I might be depressed (before the lymphoma was diagnosed). Some took me to play golf, see Lions games, and watch movies. One friend went with me to buy a new bike. Another cleared my driveway every time it snowed. Even when I was void of emotion, couldn't express myself, and couldn't even keep my balance, these guys were by my side.

Other friends tried to help by bringing me a new juicer and a recipe book full of healthy options for me to try. We received a collection of gift cards to various restaurants so we could order out instead of making dinner, which was a huge help for our busy household. Everyone tried to do something to help Keri, our family, or me. It was like we had a whole team of people helping us, holding us up, and supporting us during the darkest time.

While I rested one day, Keri replied to multiple text messages at once:

> After round five of chemo, Rob developed an awful stomachache. We thought it was either chemo side effects or the flu. When he started vomiting blood on Sunday, we knew it was something else. I took him to the Beaumont ER and he was checked in. It was his gall bladder. After the surgeons removed it, they found that it had turned completely black. The surgeon said it was one of the top three worst gall bladders he's ever seen! My parents took the kids for the week so I could be with him while he was in the hospital. Michele, Cindy, and Rob's parents waited with me during his surgery, for moral support. As always, we thank all of you for your prayers. We're back home now, and Rob is resting. Round six of chemo has been pushed back a couple weeks to give him time to recuperate a bit. I'll keep you all updated, and thank you again for your calls and prayers.

After round six of chemo, I was once again scheduled for radiation at Beaumont, although Dr. Junck had some reservations about me doing it. We trusted him, so we wanted to hear what he had to say. He told us, "There are some possible cognitive side effects. Let me look into it and give it some thought about how we should proceed."

Keri and I weren't thrilled about having my brain irradiated, so we were glad the doctor wanted to look into it further. We trusted his opinion.

Before long, we all decided I should go ahead and do the radiation, but we'd do the minimum number of treatments and the minimum dosage of radiation. It was a full-head treatment, but each session lasted only three minutes. The radiation was harder on me this time, and I ended up doing twelve out of a possible fifteen sessions.

On my last day of radiation, since we'd previously learned of the significance of the bell ceremony, the whole family came to watch me ring the bell and celebrate the end of my treatment. Keri and the boys were there, as were my parents, Keri's parents, my sister, and my brother-in-law. Afterward, we all went out to brunch together. But my energy had been entirely sapped, as if the life had been drained from my body. I just wanted to get home and rest.

During the three weeks after my final radiation treatment, I was so weak and so tired I thought I might die. I had zero energy; I couldn't articulate words that were in my head; and I still couldn't relate to my old world. Keri constantly helped me, doing things for me like bringing me water or more blankets. Even the simple task of daily showers was completely exhausting. I'd be in the shower for an hour as the water ran over me, but I was too weak to shampoo myself. Keri even had to help me to put on my socks and underwear.

My skin looked like a colorful, peeling mosaic, all in various stages of healing. The itchiness was excruciating. I could hardly stand it; I felt like I wanted to itch myself from the inside out. While I didn't like how I *looked*, my outward appearance wasn't nearly as awful as how I *felt* inside. *Exhausted* was an understatement.

During this time, I couldn't even verbalize Max's name. He's my dad's namesake, and his middle name is also Keri's father's name. The only thing worse than the constant fatigue was the frightening frustration that also plagued me. "I can't do this anymore," I told Keri one day. "It's like I beat the cancer with chemo, but now the radiation is going to take me out."

"You'll get past it," she reassured me. "You will. Just get through one day at a time."

Go! Go! Go! I silently reminded myself.

Just when I thought I could take no more, I began to feel the slightest bit better. It was also nearly time for me to see Dr. Junck for a follow-up visit.

11
Rise

By Calla

Keri drove me to my appointment with Dr. Junck. But first he had scheduled me for an MRI, so I went to radiology before we saw him. I used to be claustrophobic, but I had trained myself to forget the anxiety I felt in small spaces. I listened to music and cleared my mind while the noisy machine went to work. Keri and I met with Dr. Junck an hour or so after the MRI.

"Rob, I want to do a few simple memory tests with you," he said. "Just basic stuff to check cognitive and balance reactions."

"Okay, sure."

"I'd like you to remember these three words: *Ohio, cat, shoe.*"

"Okay, sure. No problem."

Dr. Junck went on to talk about general things, like the weather and our boys. The atmosphere was light, and he and I talked briefly.

"Now, Rob," the doctor said, about five minutes later, "What were those three words I asked you to remember?"

The words. The three words. What were they? My mind raced

103

and searched to recall those three simple words. It had been only a few minutes since he'd told me to remember them.

I glanced at Keri, seated beside me, as she bit her bottom lip, looked at me, and silently willed me to recall the three simple words.

Surely I can remember something so simple!

I wracked my brain and quickly became frustrated. I could *see* the words and even *spell* them, but I couldn't *articulate* them. "I can't!" I blurted out as my palms sweat and my heart raced. "I can't recall the words!"

Keri put her hand on my arm to reassure me.

"It's all right, Rob," Dr. Junck said. "It's early still. Give it some time. Sometimes it takes a while for the neural cognitive impairments to repair themselves. Let's move on to a few other tests."

He asked me to walk up and down the hall while he watched and made notes. I couldn't keep my balance and was unable to walk in a straight line. He intently watched and made notes. Then he asked me to balance on just the balls of my feet and then squat with my hands held out in front of me. It was obvious to all of us that my ability to keep my balance had been affected. The doctor made more notes, and then he tested the strength of my handgrip and my pull-push abilities. I was unable to push back against his hands, and most notably, I couldn't make my hands roll as the doctor had asked. It was awkward and frightening not to be able to do the simple tasks as directed.

"Good. Okay, that's good," Dr. Junck said as he wrote on his chart. "I'd like for you to start speech therapy and physical therapy, Rob. We'll get it set up for you, and someone will call you about the dates. Speech therapy will help you with recall, and with physical therapy, you'll begin to see improvements, little by little, in your balance and flexibility."

Keri had been raised in a Catholic home, and our boys were Catholic. I'd considered converting to Catholicism before. Now, more than ever, I felt I needed something more to hang onto. I needed to have the strength of something bigger than me, something omnipotent that could bear the burden of all I was feeling.

In August 2014 I began the process of converting to Catholicism. I also started physical therapy around that time. It felt right to me that I should work on my physical self and my spiritual self at the same time. Renewing and revitalizing my whole self became my mission, and I delved into the process full force, just as I would have taken on a project at work. I did research, read, made plans, set goals, and measured and recorded my progress. Rebuilding Rob became my job, and I was determined to come back better and stronger than before cancer had interrupted my life and upended my family's world.

Physical therapy was sometimes difficult, but even the worst days were made better by the wonderful people at the therapy offices. The therapists helped me improve my balance and work on my flexibility. We worked toward having me walk erect, and we corrected the shuffling that had become my signature gait. But my shoulder still drooped.

It took about six months for me to relearn many simple, basic things I'd done without thinking for four decades. It was truly humbling to realize I was working on things so simple, things I'd taken for granted my whole life.

My physical therapy was made more difficult by the fact that I'd gotten out of shape in the last year, as I'd been concentrating on battling cancer. I was overweight, but I was also bloated due to the steroids I'd been taking. I wasn't happy with my appearance, and I knew getting in shape would make me feel better both physically and mentally.

My therapists, Heather and Karen, were sensitive to my physical state as they helped me work at my own pace until I'd finally built up some endurance and strength again. Their positive attitudes, compassion, and friendliness pulled me through some really rough times. They were there to work not only on my physical needs but also my whole being while they worked with me.

Whenever I felt like giving up, I silently reminded myself, *Go! Go! Go!* as I repeatedly vowed to *kick cancer's ass*. That simple phrase, "Go! Go! Go!" became my mantra, and before long, the therapists were repeating it. "Come on, Rob!" they'd cheer. "Go! Go! Go! Two more reps!" Or "Go! Go! Go! You've got this, Rob!" And "One more lap, Rob! *Go! Go! Go!*"

In addition to the physical therapists, a trainer at my gym helped me to learn the various machines and how to use them correctly for optimum results. As I got stronger physically and fed my soul spiritually, I felt myself evolving and growing.

My life seemed to be divided into two segments: my first life, *before* cancer, and my second life, *after* cancer. My first life in the fast-paced corporate world had been one of pressures, deadlines, projects, and endless workdays that merged one into the next. I had worked diligently to provide *for* my family, but I was so overworked that I didn't get to be *with* my family. I contributed to the big picture, but I never had time for the details or the little moments that made up that marvelous big picture—and our boys were growing up fast.

In my second life, my world slowed down against my will. I was no longer on the outside looking in and seeing the big picture. I was *inside* the big picture, an integral and hands-on part of it, as I navigated the intricacies of our family life.

With Keri back to work, I'd begun to help with some of the parenting duties. She still got the boys ready for school in the mornings, did the laundry, and cooked dinner, but I took them to the bus stop and drove them to practices to help as much as I could. It felt good when it was sometimes Dad the boys called for when they fell off a skateboard, needed help with their homework, or required a referee. It felt good to have them rely on me and reach out for me once in a while, instead of viewing me only as the busy parent whose cell phone was eternally attached to his head.

"You know," I told Keri one night, "I had no idea what I was missing out on all those years. And the boys really like having you at home too. You're getting to know them on another level. You'd have missed out on so much. It's like the silver lining in what you've been through in the last couple years."

Keri and I had lots of talks when I was able to speak again, and

I made sure she knew how much she'd contributed to my positive outcome. She was the rock that held me up, both figuratively and physically. We both learned something about ourselves as well as each other during the darkest time of our lives.

I learned that I couldn't have found a better wife than Keri, and our boys couldn't have a better mother. Not only did she bear an immense burden and take charge of our whole life, but she also became my advocate, making difficult decisions when I wasn't able. Many times I've reflected on our marriage vows—"for better or for worse and in sickness or in health"—and realized the intensity and depth of our promises to one another.

As I continued with my Catholic conversion, I prayed more, and I repeatedly thanked God for all the good things I had in my life. I was working hard to recover from what my body had been put through, and I felt like one of the luckiest and most blessed guys on earth.

12

Alive and Amplified

By The Mooney Suzuki

My second life, as I like to refer to it, means that I had to learn some things—a lot of things, really. In my first life, I was always the guy who arrived home after dark to a nicely manicured lawn—because I'd hired a lawn service, since I never had time to care for it myself. Today Max handles that responsibility and happily mows it with his new riding mower.

When Keri and I were first married, the only thing I knew how to cook was from a can marked "Chef Boyardee." I'll never cook like Keri, and I think we're all happier to leave most of the cooking to her, but my mom has been teaching me to cook a few things. While I used to be a great delegator, today I try to be more participative and hands-on with things. Keri and I have created systems that work for both of us and for the boys, again representative of the give-and-take that's found in marriages.

Over the past twenty-eight years, I've been to more concerts than I can even count. Music has always been very important to me, and I have the biggest CD collection of anyone I've met, with thousands neatly lining the shelves in my home office. During my first life, Keri and I went to concerts only in the Detroit area because of my work schedule, but once I wasn't working, we had more flexibility.

"This will be the Year of the Concerts!" I proclaimed in early 2014. Keri and I went to concerts in four states that year: Michigan, Ohio, Illinois, and Nevada. We went to a three-day music festival in Chicago with friends. We flew to Las Vegas to see one of our favorite bands, Jane's Addiction. We drove to Cleveland to see the Rock & Roll Hall of Fame and attend a concert. The next day, we drove to Columbus to see another show.

I was still a bit weak and couldn't stand for long periods, so Keri and I got seats in the venues' handicapped areas. And even this was a plus because we were much closer to the stages. Again, there was a silver lining.

We'd decided to have as many adventures as possible and to live life to the fullest. We took the kids to Myrtle Beach; took two trips to Las Vegas—one to renew our wedding vows; went to Mackinac Island with my in-laws; took the kids to Chicago; and spent a month at Lake of the Ozarks. Every day was a blessing and gift, and we were determined to get as much out of life as possible.

After I survived my second bout with cancer, everything seemed more meaningful and important. The sky seemed bluer, flowers smelled sweeter, and my wife's smile seemed broader. I'd always appreciated our families, but after my ordeal, they meant even more to me. Dad and I haven't missed a Detroit Lions game since 1996, no matter how sick I was, and I look forward to carrying on the father-son tradition with each of my boys. Even the simplest things hold deeper meaning, and I am grateful for each one.

As much as I loved being part of the boys' lives on a more intimate level, it bothered me that I wasn't fulfilling my traditional role as our family's main provider. In time, as I got stronger, I put out some feelers and looked into finding a job again.

At almost forty-three and having been out of the workforce for a while, getting a new job wasn't as easy as it once had been. It was very difficult to me to be considered for positions that were well below the level I'd attained in my first life. At Hydeswort, only a handful of executives had risen to the same level as I. I knew that major retailers usually have only four employees at that level within their organizations, so my odds of landing a similar position weren't good.

In the past, I'd been sought out and offered positions based on my reputation and previous performance in the industry. I liked that guy, whose reputation preceded him and whose work ethic was well known. It's who I was, and my professional identity told me how and where I fit into the world. In my second life, I felt like a puzzle piece trying to find where I fit. The whole business of looking for a job was new to me.

Just before Hydeswort let me go, I'd brought on a new employee named Belinda. Imagine my surprise when I learned that as soon as they fired me, Hydeswort gave my job to her. Of course, I spent the next couple years feeling she was an adversary of a sort.

Hydeswort let Belinda go a year after they fired me, and she became a representative for a company based in Fort Wayne, Indiana. By the time our paths crossed again, she was the executive vice president of business development for IDS.

"Rob!" Belinda said when I called, "I've wondered how you've been doing!" Her attitude was so positive and her voice so friendly, it perplexed me, since I thought she'd essentially taken my job at Hydeswort. But as we talked, I realized things weren't at all as they seemed.

"I thought I'd be working with *you* when Hydeswort hired me," Belinda told me. "I was really mad and totally shocked when they let you go. No one saw it coming."

I'd spent the past couple years having bad feelings for no reason at all. Things weren't as I'd imagined, and I'd wasted my time and energy dwelling on something that wasn't at all as I'd thought.

After we talked a few times, Belinda hired me as vice president of business development, the position I'd held at Hydeswort. Better still was the fact that I could work from home in my new position. If things hadn't all fallen into place as they did, I'd never have had the opportunity to work with such a high-quality person in such a great organization. Things happen for a reason.

With my health improving and my new job, things were definitely looking up. But something had been bothering me for well over a year. It kept me up some nights and occupied my mind as unfinished business. I hadn't resolved things with Bruce at Hydeswort, and I've never been the kind of guy to leave things undone. I had to resolve how I'd been treated and what had been done to me. The fact that Hydeswort had settled out of court with me was sort of a resolution in itself, but I needed a personal conclusion. It was something I had to do once and for all to close the final chapter on my first life.

After considering what I wanted to say to Bruce, I called him one afternoon. Because I was still having some memory issues and difficulty recalling how to say certain words, I planned to stay focused and to get right to the point of my call.

"Rob Atteberry!" Bruce said when he took my call. "How are you doing?"

"I need to talk to you, Bruce."

"Okay, sure. Come on down to the office."

I went to the corporate offices and was buzzed into the second floor, where Bruce's office was. "I'll get Bruce for you," the receptionist told me.

Moments later, Bruce came out of the boardroom, and we shook hands and exchanged pleasantries. "We can step in here," he soon said, and I followed him into the boardroom.

After we sat down, I looked him in the eye, and said, "Bruce, I am going to talk to you. I do not want you to talk. This is what I'm here to tell you: I came to work here back in 2012 because you were my mentor and I wanted to work for you again. I was doing well, but then I got cancer, and you let me go. That was a problem. I put off my radiation treatments because I thought I no longer had insurance. My cancer ended up coming back in my brain.

"It's a long and intense story, but thanks to my family and friends, I got through it. Little by little, I grew stronger, learned to walk and talk again and to be a husband and a father again. But through it all, I wondered how to explain to my kids that their father had no job. I'm here today to tell you to look in the mirror, Bruce. Don't ever repeat what you did to me. Don't put someone else through the hell that you put me through. And by the way, I'm in remission now."

Bruce didn't look at me for much of what I said to him. He looked down and hung his head slightly as I spoke. I wondered if he'd expected to hear from me and even if he felt he deserved to be admonished like a child.

When I'd finished speaking, Bruce took a deep breath and looked up. "Congratulations," he said almost robotically.

"Thank you," I calmly said. "I'm going to leave now."

I got up and walked out of the boardroom and through the door. As I walked through the lobby, I felt a little bit lighter.

"Hey, Rob!" Bruce called behind me. "Rob, wait a minute."

I turned around, and Bruce walked up to me.

"You know, Bruce, I was a vice president for you at Gechsmin; I was a vice president at Tendlart and then a vice president for you *again* at Hydeswort. You could've put me on disability, but you fired me. Things could have been different and so much easier."

"I know" was all he said.

Shaking my head, I turned my back on him, but this time,

I kept walking. I wondered if he had so little to say because the legal department had told him not to discuss the matter with me or anyone else. Nonetheless, I felt great when I walked out of the building that day. As the door closed behind me, I knew I had also closed the final chapter of my first life, and I felt satisfied.

That night, I easily fell asleep and slept better than I had in a long time. When the sun came up the next morning, it brought with it the promise of good things in my second life, and I was ready to embrace all of them.

13
True Faith

By New Order

As life started looking up for me, I realized I was growing and becoming a different person in a lot of ways. I looked at life differently, and I valued my life and the people in it more. Instead of being constantly distracted and having a cell phone plastered to my ear all the time, I embraced everyone and everything in my life, and I thanked God for all the blessings around me, big and small. Instead of being distracted and in a hurry all the time, I slowed down to enjoy the little things, like stealing a kiss from my wife at a stoplight or getting caught in the rain while we were out for a walk. Instead of being irritated that the dog's toys were on the floor, I was grateful that I could walk over and pick them up. Instead of immediately becoming stressed over situations, I reminded myself how awesome it is to *be here* to deal with those situations. I saw things differently and in a new light. Compared to what I'd been through, life looked pretty good to me.

It was spring 2015, and I was nearing the end of my conversion to Catholicism. (Coincidentally, my Cobra insurance coverage was nearing its end too.) During a six-hour sabbatical with Father Mike in March, he related a story to me. He told me of a twenty-seven-year-old, good-looking guy who had a million dollars and found out he had cancer.

"So what did he do?" I asked.

"Well, he took all his money and went to Florida," Father Mike said.

"And?"

"*And he died*. He didn't ask for God's help; he didn't seek guidance; and he didn't try to save himself. Instead he died with a full bank account and an empty heart."

"You know, Father Mike, I had cancer," I said. "But now I'm in remission. It was a combination of things—family, friends, fitness, the doctors—that helped, but I know God is the reason I'm still here."

"Well, I'm certain of it," Father Mike said.

When my thirty-month Cobra coverage ended on March 31, 2015, I was forced to go on Medicare. Keri and the boys are covered under Obamacare. I really resent that Hydeswort never gave me the opportunity to go on disability. Instead they chose to sever my employment and effectively throw my world and my family's world into a tailspin. Life was made so much more difficult as a result, and the stress was compounded tenfold because of the company's irresponsible decisions and inhumane actions.

A few days before my Cobra coverage ended, I sat down in front of my computer and opened my Facebook page. There were the usual new posts, and then I saw a familiar name in the comments section under an update I'd posted about my good MRI scan.

Steve Ryman was my indirect boss years when I was with Gechsmin. Seeing his name reminded me of the great guy he was and how he'd been so supportive during my cancer battle.

"Freaking fantastic news about your PET scan!" he wrote on March 27. "You've *got* to write a book! Now get going on it! You'll make a million dollars!"

I laughed aloud at Steve's comment, "liked" it, and went on to read other Facebook posts. Just five days later, I got devastating news: Steve had committed suicide. As I talked with people, it became clear that due to his own medical problems and his dismal prognosis, he had decided when and how he'd leave this life. He had lost sight in one eye and was rapidly losing sight in the other. Steve had never married and had no kids, so I presumed he just didn't want to live without his sight.

When I heard the awful news, I went to Steve's Facebook page and saw the familiar photos of him with his beloved horses and dogs. Everyone who knew him also knew how much he loved animals. He gave of himself and always helped others. He was a great guy, loved and respected by so many. And just as he'd always been in charge of his life, Steve also made the decision, at age fifty-nine, to check out on his own terms and in his own time. He'd even left instructions that he have no funeral or service of any kind.

It seemed bizarre to me that I was fighting with everything I had to live and to stay here with Keri and our boys, but Steve had chosen to leave this world. I reasoned that he must have made the best decision for himself and his circumstances, just as I'd done. I prayed for Steve and even talked to him, telling him we'd meet again one day—but not too soon, if I had anything to say about it.

After Steve's death, I vowed to lead a full and valuable life. I realized that even in death, Steve continued to inspire me. And his final Facebook message to me prompted me to share my own journey with others.

Just a few days later, on Easter Sunday, I completed my conversion to Catholicism. That day held special meaning for me as I embraced not only my second life but also my deeper relationship with God. I was new, healthy, and whole that day, and I was grateful to be here with my family.

As great as life looked for me, I didn't forget that many others still suffered with cancer and the collateral damage it leaves. I'd become active in Gilda's Club, both for me and for other cancer patients and their families.

The original chapter of Gilda's Club was formed in New York and named for Gilda Radner, the brilliant comedian and an original cast member of *Saturday Night Live*. Even after Gilda was diagnosed with ovarian cancer in 1986, she continued to make people laugh, and she learned to live with her cancer. It was her dream that all people touched by cancer receive the social and emotional support she'd found during her battle.

After she lost her battle in 1989, her husband, Gene Wilder, and her cancer psychotherapist formed the first Gilda's Club. Six years later, the New York City chapter officially opened its doors, and the members poured in through the group's signature red door, which represents Gilda's legacy to those living with cancer.

Gilda's Club is intended to be a gathering place where cancer patients and their families go to find social and emotional support as a supplement to medical care. Nearly fifteen million people are diagnosed with cancer each year, and many rely on their Gilda's Club meetings. They look forward to passing through the red door and finding understanding, solace, and hope on the other side.

Since I'd beaten cancer twice, I resolved to be a beacon of hope for people in the battle of their lives and for their very lives. My involvement with Gilda's Club led me to meet some incredible people, and my eyes were opened to the fact that a lot of cancer patients don't have as much support as I had during my own cancer fights. Many of the cancer patients couldn't afford the chemotherapy recommended by their doctors, so their visits to Gilda's Club were the only medicine they received.

We all had different stories, different circumstances, and other things that separated us, yet we shared our battle with cancer. I made an effort to connect with people and to offer them hope at these groups. Attending the meetings was very intense and emotionally draining; I'd even feel exhausted through the next day. But since I'd beaten cancer not once but twice, I owed it to others to be a living example of someone who had made it out the other side and defeated the monster that they battled.

In addition to sharing our health issues and our personal experiences, the group members shared personal problems and stories of our own insurance woes. It was obvious that while we all shared similarities, we also had different dynamics at play in our personal lives. For me, my health had become a top priority, so I decided to focus on preparing for an upcoming triathlon as a way to stay focused.

With everything going on in 2014, it was important that I had a goal, something to work toward, a deadline of sorts that would measure my progress. Maybe that mind-set was formed during my days in the corporate world, but I'm a guy who enjoys that sort of thing, thriving in that atmosphere. So I was determined to complete the September 2014 Reeds Lake Triathlon.

In 2009, the Reeds Lake Tri had been my first. Years later, after all I'd been through, I wanted to do it again to prove to myself that I was indeed back. To train for the 2014 tri, I ran, biked, and swam to prepare my body for the half-mile swim, 18.5-mile bike ride, and four-mile run.

Just a couple of months after I completed speech and physical therapy, I was back at the Reeds Lake Tri with about 1,200 other athletes, each of us there for our own reasons. For years, the tri had been held to promote an active, healthy lifestyle and to raise awareness for the Mary Free Bed Rehabilitation Hospital

Foundation, which helped restore hope and freedom through rehabilitation. I was there because I'd also found hope and freedom through rehab; but I was also there to prove something to myself and to cap off the progress I'd made in recent months.

Keri trained to compete in the team relay event. She was her team's swimmer for the first part of the tri; Jill was the cyclist; and Theresa was the runner. Our friend Shannon organized two other relays of women, all wearing Team Atts shirts.

The air was full of team spirit on the most perfect Michigan days we'd had in a while, almost as if God was smiling down and rejoicing with us in my triumph over cancer. The skies were blue and clear, and the temperature was about seventy degrees. The swimmers needed wetsuits, but the temperature was perfect for the cyclists and runners.

I'd had the support of all our family and friends from the beginning of my battle with cancer, but it was amazing to see those who'd come out to support me at the triathlon. There was an endless sea of blue T-shirts emblazoned with Team Atts on the fronts and Go! Go! Go! on the backs. The presence of Team Atts energized me; the air was charged with the love and encouragement of the people who mean the most to me. I felt like a winner before I even started.

From the moment I took my first stroke in the lake's frigid water, our friend, James, was by my side; he matched his strokes to mine and never left me. His presence pushed me, stroke after stroke, as I cut through the water. When I got to the other side of the lake, I ran from the water's edge to pick up my bike, and Bob and James were right there. I was empowered by my friends' support as I pedaled for all I was worth and left cancer behind—in my past.

This is what life's all about, I thought. *This is what's important!*

Just seven months before, I'd completed my radiation treatments and had begun speech and physical therapy. The road hadn't been easy, but it was made much easier by family and friends like those on the bikes beside me. As I focused on the road in front of me, I pedaled into my future, excited for what would come next.

When I came to the end of the 18.5-mile route, I dropped my bike and began the final leg: the four-mile run. Bob and James were still right there with me, and Theresa ran with us at that point, doing her part of the relay for Keri's team. I was maintaining a run-walk pace, but our friends stayed beside me and kept pace with me, ignoring their own potential finish times.

About a mile from the finish line, another friend, Marc, ran up and joined our group. He had already completed the course, but he'd come back to run with me and encourage me as I headed for the finish line. As I focused and controlled my breathing, step after step, I felt the support of my friends as sure as if they'd carried me. They all knew how important it was for me to get to the end of the race unassisted and on my own.

"You've got this, Rob!" they said. "Almost there! You're doing great!"

Finally, the finish line came into view, roped-off with yellow tape and surrounded by orange cones and tents on either side. But it wasn't the finish line that I focused on as I made my way to the end of the race. It was the huge sea of blue T-shirts and homemade poster board signs made by Team Atts.

"Yeah, Dad! Come on, Dad!" my boys yelled from the sidelines, among the blue shirts that rose up around them.

My own sleeveless blue shirt got closer to the vast sea of blue step by step until I finally crossed the finish line. Tears in my eyes, hidden by my sunglasses, I crossed the white line with hands held high as my friends hung back and allowed me to cross alone. It was the first time in two hours that they'd left my side. Enveloped by sixty people in blue shirts that wrapped me with their love, I was reminded of how and why I'm still here and how grateful I am for this gift called life.

The applause and cheers had made my finish seem more like a major sporting event, and I'd never felt better. As weak and lifeless as I'd been just months earlier, in that moment I felt invincible—like I could move mountains! Friends and family cheered, clapped, and took photos as Keri came to kiss me. She was right there, just as she'd been from the start of my cancer battle, to support me, hold me, and lift me up.

The announcer told the crowd, "Well, I'll tell you one thing. This is the biggest cheering crew around! This is Mr. Rob Atteberry, folks. He's a Grand Rapids cancer survivor."

Yes, I am! I thought. *I surely am!*

No race had ever felt better, and no finish line had looked brighter. All our friends and family joined us for a great after-party at Marc and Shannon's house. We didn't just celebrate my completion of the tri though; we celebrated our love and friendship that day—the things that really matter.

"I want to thank each and every one you," I said in a toast, as I looked at all the faces around me, "for being so important to my family and to me and for all you do for us. Everything about the tri was important, but what's more important is *all of you* and what you mean to our family and to me. Your love and support got us through one of the roughest times in our lives. I love all of you more than I can ever say. Go! Go! Go!"

After completing the triathlon in September 2014, it was important to me to continue to get healthier and to continue to set goals for myself. I first started competing in triathlons because I'd put on some weight and I wanted to get in shape again. But after beating cancer, the triathlons meant so much more than that to me. Training, competing, and finishing triathlons allows me to set goals, work toward them, and then compete, which allows me to see my efforts pay off.

Charting and measuring my progress and my accomplishments is a visual reminder to me of how far I've come and the work I've done. Finishing a race or a triathlon doesn't mean just crossing the finish line. It means weeks and months of training that culminates in proving that I'm transforming myself and getting stronger, that I'm healthy and that I'm still here.

14
Hands Up, Robert

By Saint Motel

With life looking up and a few triathlons under my belt, my next goal was to complete the 1/2 Ironman Muncie in Muncie, Indiana, in July 2015. I'd trained religiously, paced myself, set small and then larger goals, and kept my eye on my objective. I felt great, both physically and mentally, the week of the race.

But there was another equally important event on my calendar that week. As eager as I was to complete in Muncie, I was also eager to get the MRI that my doctor had scheduled for that same week.

The mood around our home was light and fun as the day of the race approached. During church on Sunday, I thanked God for all He'd done for me that had brought me to that week. I worked at home on Monday and met with a buyer in Grand Rapids on Tuesday. Keri and I cheered the boys on during a swim meet on Wednesday, and then we dropped all of them off at Keri's parents' home so the two of us could go to Detroit and see a Morrissey concert that night. The week had been fast-paced, and it felt great to have a diverse, busy schedule and a typical family life once again.

"You know," I said as we drove to Detroit, "*This* is how it's supposed to be. *This* is how life should be."

She just smiled and held my hand tighter.

We had great seats for the concert that night. I'm not sure if it was because I was in a terrific mood or if it was simply because things looked, smelled, and sounded more intense and clear, but Morrissey was fantastic. It felt good to have Keri by my side as we enjoyed the concert together, free of the worry and the burden we'd shared. Just as she'd been beside me every step of the way during my journey through cancer, Keri was right there holding my hand that night and reminding me of what's really important.

When the concert ended, we went to a hotel in Ann Arbor to get some sleep, since my MRI was scheduled for six the next morning. Just as I'd done all week, I easily woke before our four o'clock alarm sounded. I was ready to have the MRI done and get confirmation that the prognosis was good once again.

When we arrived at the University of Michigan's cancer center, I wasn't the least bit worried that we'd hear bad news after the MRI. Keri and I thought only positive thoughts, and we went in there merely as a formality.

While completely still inside the MRI machine, I silently reminded myself, *Go! Go! Go!* The magnetic field and pulses of radio-wave energy reverberated around my head as I lay perfectly still, just as I'd done for the previous three MRIs, which had all yielded favorable results. I waited silently for the test that could detect tissue damage, signs of infection, inflammation, or cancer, though I was sure my results would be favorable.

Several hours later, Keri and I met with Jessica, Dr. Junck's physician's assistant. We were glad to see her because she had taken time off to have a baby before my treatments had ended. As we talked with her about her new baby, I was reminded that life goes on and that God is good indeed.

"Well, it's good news!" she told us happily. "Everything looks good. No changes."

Keri and I breathed sighs of relief. By that time, she and I were far beyond tears, either good or bad. We felt nothing but gratefulness, thankfulness, and sheer happiness on that morning. When Keri and I left Jessica, we hugged her and thanked her, grateful for another friend we'd made along our way. We walked outside the University of Michigan's hospital doors, and I was certain the morning sun was shining brighter than ever and that God smiled down on us.

Keri texted,

Great news everyone! Rob's MRI results were good!

I shared my latest good news on Facebook:

MRI WAS GOOD!!! NO CHANGES!!! GO! GO! GO!

We drove home, and while Keri went to pick up Max and Wes from their tennis matches, I drove over to her parents' home to pick up Zac and Ben. It felt great to be doing the simple Dad duties that I might have missed out on if things had turned out differently. I knew I wouldn't be here if I didn't have a persistent wife who had fought for doctors to look harder and delve deeper only months before. We were eager to set out on our trip, and I couldn't wait to celebrate life when I completed the 1/2 Ironman Muncie.

The next morning, Friday, we piled all the boys into our Suburban and set off for the four-hour drive to Muncie. As on all our family car trips, the boys were buckled in back with their travel necessities, including videos, iPads, music, books, games, and snacks.

As I drove along, I enjoyed listening to the boys joking and playing as Keri sat beside me. When I was a busy, successful executive, I thought I had it all. Now I was certain I'd been very wrong. As I looked next to me and then into the rearview mirror, I realized that *now* I have it all.

We got up early on Saturday morning, and I was eager to head over to the Prairie Creek Reservoir, located on more than 750 acres and about five miles southeast of Muncie. After 141 days of training, I felt ready to take on the challenge of the 70.3 miles that awaited me.

My cheering section was ready too, all wearing their familiar "Go! Go! Go!" blue shirts. My parents, Cindy, and her kids, and some family friends had come to support me and to wait while I competed in all three events. My longtime friend, James, was there too. He had signed up to compete alongside me and make sure I made it through the race safely.

Of the two thousand people who signed up, 1,760 competed

that day. There were men and women of all different shapes, sizes, and ages. There were some handicapped participants too.

Keri and our kids sat by the water's edge and watched as I joined the other competitors in the first event, a 1.2-mile swim across a lake. Hands and feet rhythmically sliced through the water all around me as I swam hard and remained focused. It was reassuring to see James swimming alongside of me.

Go! Go! Go! I reminded myself. *Go! Go! Go!*

I'd trained in a swimming pool, but I still did well in the open water. I finished the swim in forty minutes to place one-hundredth out of three hundred competitors in my age group—not bad for a guy who couldn't even stand without toppling just a year before.

I hurriedly got out of the lake and ran to the next event, the fifty-six-mile bike ride. My body felt great. The endorphins pulsed through me as I concentrated on the road in front of me and paced myself. I wasn't hurting at all. In fact, I felt exhilarated as James and I raced through rural Indiana. I knew the upcoming run would be tough, but I put the thought out of my mind and focused only on the task at hand as I concentrated on the road in front of me.

Go! Go! Go!

When I finished mile fifty-six, I dropped my bike and immediately began the 13.1-mile run around the south side of the reservoir, over rolling country roads, and then back again. As I ran, I was grateful to my Oakhurst Wolfpack running buddies, who had faithfully trained with me in all kinds of weather. Come rain or come shine and in all kinds of temperatures, they'd been there for me every day. I'd expected that the run would be tough, especially after the first two events, but I knew I was well prepared.

James ran beside me in case I needed something. I appreciated having him there, and he played an integral part in me finishing that day. It helped to have someone to keep pace with and to strategize with as our strides fell into step and I mirrored mine to his. James and I had decided I should run the first eight miles and then walk fast and jog the last couple miles to come in under the allotted time.

When overwhelming fatigue caused my legs to have a mind of their own, James forced me to stop and drink. When I felt overwhelmed and foggy because of the fatigue, and I seemed a bit off to him, he forced me to talk so I'd have to focus again.

I ran the first eight miles and then slowed down to a fast walk, as James and I had planned. There weren't many people along the road at that point in the run, but I saw one man standing at the road's edge up ahead in the distance.

"Ryan?" I yelled out when we made eye contact. "Ryan Shepherd?! What are you doing here?"

"I saw on Facebook that you'd be here today, so I figured I'd come out and support you," he said as he also fell in step beside me. "I called Cindy and told her I'd be waiting for you along the route."

"You drove over an hour just to come out here for *me*?" I asked. "Man, I haven't seen you in *fifteen years*. That's so incredible!"

"Of course! I wouldn't miss it," Ryan said. "I was surprised no one stopped me when I walked out near the course, but here I am."

I was very touched by yet another friend's support. It was amazing to me that he was out there. "Sorry, I can't talk too much," I told him as I measured my breathing. "We can talk at the end."

"No problem. I understand. I'll be right here beside you though."

As Ryan, James, and I walked and ran, a woman came up beside me. "Mind if I run with you?" she asked as she focused on the route in front of us.

"Not at all."

I tried not to talk much and to preserve my energy, but she talked to me as we began to run again at mile eleven. She explained that she'd needed someone to run with so she could make it to the finish line.

"I'm doing this race to honor my baby," she explained. "The baby I lost at five months."

"Wow, I'm really sorry," I offered as my heart broke for her.

"Thanks."

She and I continued on, each focused and lost in our own thoughts, but each still keeping pace with the other. I realized all the race participants had their own reasons for being out there on that day. Those reasons were as varied and diverse as their own life stories. Even as different as the participants were, each of us focused on the same finish line.

As we approached mile marker twelve, James said he'd run ahead and tell my family and friends I was coming. He sprinted ahead.

Go! Go! Go! I thought as I waved him on. *Go! Go! Go!*

James ran back to me again minutes later and was matching his steps with mine. Just before we got close to the finish line, Ryan and James veered off the course and let me run the last half mile or so on my own.

"See ya at the finish line!" they yelled, and I waved and smiled without speaking.

As I put one foot in front of the other, I thought of all I'd been through in the last couple of years. So much had led up to that very moment. While I was about to cross the finish line, I knew it really marked the *beginning* of the rest of my life and all the goodness that was yet to come. As I measured my breathing and kept running, I thanked God that I was still here and able to take a breath.

Suddenly I heard cheering and clapping and saw a huge inflatable marker in the distance. There was a sea of blue Team Atts T-shirts worn by my friends and family and a bunch of homemade signs and banners. As everyone clapped and cheered, people shook cowbells and yelled for me as I got closer and closer to my goal. With my arms over my head, I ran across the finish line with six minutes to spare.

An official came over and hung a medal around my neck as my family and friends clapped, yelled, and cheered. I walked a bit more so my leg muscles wouldn't cramp, and then I went over and hugged everyone. They all thought they were celebrating me and my feat, but it was really *I* who celebrated *them* and all they meant to me.

Soaking wet from head to toe, with sweat running down my body and my heart still pumping hard, I tried to catch my breath.

It felt great that I'd completed the Half Ironman, and even with time to spare. But as I looked at all the faces around me, young and old, I knew why my heart was so full, and it had nothing to do with the last 70.3 miles.

EPILOGUE

After the Half Ironman in Muncie, we celebrated with family and friends. Then Keri and I decided to get a hotel room for the night and drive home in the morning. Needless to say, the boys were happy to extend our family's adventure. As we all fell asleep that night, I thanked God for getting me to where I was in life and for giving me the five gifts that make my life worth living.

On the Monday afternoon following the Half Ironman, I posted an update to my Facebook page as always:

> Quick update! Today was Day 1 of 63 days of training for the Reed's Lake Triathlon!
>
> *~ Well, you didn't think I was going to STOP, did you? ~*
> *Kicking Cancers A**!!!*
> *GO! GO! GO!!!*

GO! GO! GO! PLAYLIST:
MUSIC THAT INSPIRED THE BOOK

1. To Be Young," Ryan Adams
2. Begin the Begin," REM
3. "I'm Ready," Twin Shadows
4. "Something's Wrong," Sloan
5. "Seasons," Future Islands
6. "Running up that Hill," Kate Bush
7. "The Way We Get By," Spoon
8. "A Pain That I'm Used To," Depeche Mode
9. "Everything Is Wrong," Interpol
10. "Clinically Dead," Chad VanGaalen
11. "Rise," Calla
12. "Alive and Amplified," Mooney Suzuki
13. "True Faith," New Order
14. "Hands Up, Robert," Saint Motel

Listen to "Go! Go! Go! Rise, Fall, and Rise Again" at https://itunes. apple.com/us/playlist/go!go!go!-rise-fall-rise-again/idpl.07afaa55fd 334c91a6256b77e0532914.

Printed in the United States
By Bookmasters

Printed in the United States
By Bookmasters